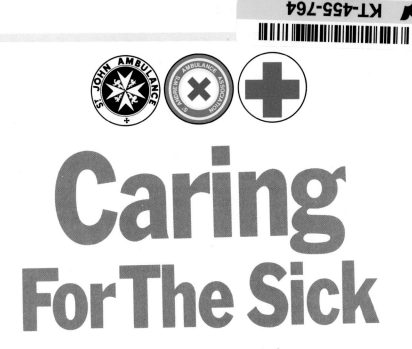

Caring
For The Sick

The Authorised Manual of
St. John Ambulance
St. Andrew's Ambulance Association
The British Red Cross Society

Dorling Kindersley · London

All enquiries regarding any extracts or re-use of any
material in this book should be addressed to the
publishers Dorling Kindersley Ltd.

Second edition first published in Great Britain in 1988 by
Dorling Kindersley Limited, 9 Henrietta Street,
Covent Garden, London WC2E 8PS.

First impression September 1988
Conjoint Societies 50,000 copies
Trade 5,000 copies

Second impression December 1990
Conjoint Societies 30,000 copies
Trade 5,000 copies

Third impression July 1993
Trade 6,000 copies
Fourth impression June 1995
Trade 4,000 copies

British Library Cataloguing in Publication Data

Caring for the sick.
1. Sick Persons. Care
I. St. John Ambulance Association and
Brigade II. St. Andrew's Ambulance
Association III. Red Cross. *British Red
Cross Society*
362.1

ISBN 0–86318–320–4

Caring
For The Sick

CONTENTS

CONTENTS

ELIMINATION: Helping the patient to deal with his excretions — 82

REST AND SLEEP: Helping the patient to relax and maintain good sleeping habits — 99

CONTROLLING TEMPERATURE: Helping the patient to maintain normal body temperature — 104

CARING FOR A WOUND: Helping the patient with an injury — 116

BREATHING DIFFICULTIES: Helping the patient to breathe more easily — 126

COMMUNICATION: Helping the patient to communicate his needs effectively — 134

CONTENTS

THE VOLUNTARY AID SOCIETIES

THE ST JOHN AMBULANCE

The Order of St John of Jerusalem can be traced back to times before the Great Crusades, when the brothers tended pilgrims on their way to Jerusalem. Today it still has two great Foundations: the Ophthalmic Hospital in Jerusalem, and the Ambulance, which has two branches, the Association, responsible for training, and the Brigade, whose uniforms are so familiar at public functions. In any one year the Brigade carries out more than four million hours of duties. The local unit of the Brigade is the Division; here the members meet together each week to undergo training in first aid and nursing. Doctors and nurses who are also members of the Brigade meet with them to teach and supervise their practice. The junior branch, the Cadets (10–16 year olds), take part in many outdoor activities as well as nursing, first aid and child care. The Badgers (6–10 year olds) have a simple course in "absolutely everything". The picture shows the uniform adult members of the Brigade wear when performing nursing duties, either at home or in hospital.

ST ANDREW'S AMBULANCE ASSOCIATION

St Andrew's Ambulance Association was founded in Glasgow in 1882, created by the joint efforts of the city's medical profession, community interests and business and industry in a welfare initiative which was far ahead of its time.

Today, after over a century of caring, that commitment to community welfare remains the keystone of the Association's work. It is one of Scotland's largest charities, concentrating its efforts on training its own members, and many others from all walks of life, in first aid, caring for the sick and the injured, and other health and welfare matters. Members of the Association's Corps of volunteers are familiar figures in Scotland, at events ranging from football internationals to Royal visits. Less visible but just as important is the help given, week in and week out, to countless smaller local events, aiding the chronically ill, the handicapped and the elderly.

That service, together with its training programmes, keeps the community commitment strong.

THE BRITISH RED CROSS SOCIETY

If the British Red Cross Society did not exist, the country would be £30 million poorer. That is the value which has been put on the voluntary, unpaid, work members do each year. The Society, which has branches throughout the UK, is not government funded and relies on voluntary contributions. It trains its members, and members of the public, in first aid, nursing, and other community services. Members work to alleviate suffering among sick, injured, handicapped and elderly people. Our adult nursing courses take the fear and worry out of caring for a relative at home. The British Red Cross, which is non-political and non-religious, is part of the International Red Cross, the world's largest voluntary organization for the relief of pain and suffering. The picture shows the uniform members wear for nursing duties.

The British Red Cross Society

The St John Ambulance

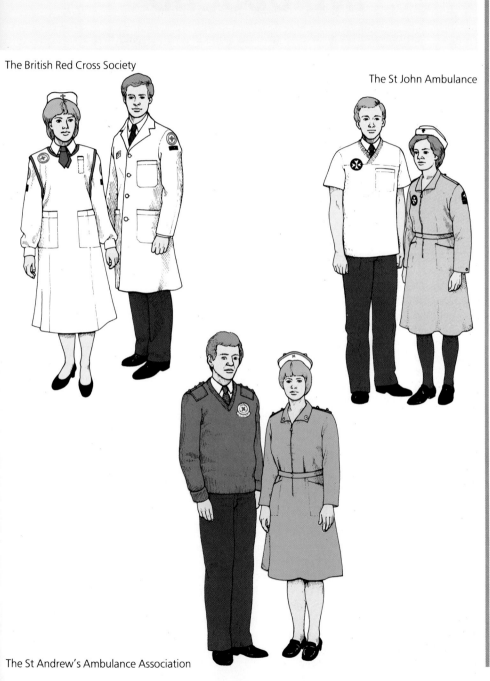

The St Andrew's Ambulance Association

INTRODUCTION

Before you undertake to give nursing care you should first ask yourself: what is nursing? It *could* be defined merely as a set of tasks to be carried out in the shortest possible time, without considering individual likes or wants. In reality, nursing is the act of looking after an individual, helping him to do what he would do by himself if he could, and helping him in such a way that he does not lose his dignity and is encouraged to regain as much independence as he can, and as soon as he can.

THE NEEDS OF THE PATIENT

The patient has the same needs as the person who is well. As you may have to help him do things that he cannot do for himself, you should know what the individual's basic needs are. Everyone needs:
■ to be in a safe environment
■ to move and maintain a comfortable position
■ to keep his body clean and well-groomed and protect his skin
■ to select suitable clothing and dress and undress
■ to eat and drink adequately
■ to eliminate
■ to sleep and rest
■ to maintain normal body temperature
■ to breathe normally
■ to communicate and express emotions, needs and fears
■ to work at something that provides a sense of accomplishment
■ to play or participate in various forms of recreation
■ to learn, discover or satisfy the curiosity that is part of normal development and health
■ to worship according to his faith.

Each of these needs should be considered in relation to the individual patient and you should ask yourself certain questions:
■ What can the patient do unaided?
■ Is his present disability temporary or permanent?
■ Can he be taught or re-taught to do the things he is unable to do at present and so gain independence?
■ If he cannot gain independence, can his family or friends help and, if so, will they require instruction?
■ Is professional help necessary through members of the health or social work teams?

If you try to answer these questions for yourself, you will be learning a great deal about the individual patient's needs. In planning individual care you must then do all you can to ensure that the physical, psychological, social, financial and spiritual needs of the individual are met.

PHYSICAL NEEDS

Physical needs include: being able to breathe, to eat and drink, to rest and sleep and to be safe in a stable environment. As you plan a daily routine for the patient you take account of these needs. You make sure he is washed, fed, gets enough sleep and stays secure in familiar surroundings. If the patient has to enter hospital, he may find that environment unfamiliar and unsettling, even hostile, in which case you need to do as much as you can to make him feel comfortable and at ease.

PSYCHOLOGICAL NEEDS

Basic psychological needs include: the need to be esteemed; the need to be valued, accepted and recognized as an individual; and the need for security and privacy. You can help to maintain the patient's self-esteem by encouraging as much independence as possible and by using a proper name and title. Many an elderly spinster feels annoyed and humiliated by being referred to as "gran". Take into account the patient's age, background, physical and mental condition and, depending on how well you know him, adjust your approach accordingly.

Ensure that privacy is available whenever the patient requires it, particularly if you are attending to his personal needs or if he wishes to talk quietly with a friend, lawyer or priest. Be alert to his feelings of insecurity, particularly if his illness has lasted for a long time and has left him severely incapacitated. Apprehension, fear and depression are often experienced by ill people.

Listen attentively to what the patient is saying; never appear hurried. Try instead to make him feel that you really care about him as a person. This is less difficult in the home than it is in a hospital or institution, where many patients are seeking your help and attention at the same time.

Young physically handicapped men and women often have sexual problems. Do not ask them questions, but if someone spontaneously confides in you let the doctor know what has been said. Psycho-sexual counselling may help not only them but their family as well and the specialists in this field are experienced and very skilled people.

SOCIAL NEEDS

Whether young or old, the patient needs companionship. Visitors are always welcome, yet they can tire the patient. Try to assess the patient's condition in order to decide how much visiting is advisable, and discuss your opinion with the family.

Radio or television can provide companionship, but sets should be placed where they can be seen easily, heard without difficulty and switched off when not required. Turning off a television set some distance away can pose a problem: a set with remote control may be the answer. Alternatively, you should make sure that you are frequently available to respond to the patient's needs.

Children confined to bed for a long period may need to continue their education. Encourage parents to consult the head teacher of the child's school as he will give advice and can make any necessary arrangements.

FINANCIAL NEEDS

Many patients are worried about money and do not realize that they may be entitled to certain pensions or allowances. The community nursing sister can give advice or you can consult the local social security office or Citizens' Advice Bureau. The Department of Health and Social Security produces leaflets explaining entitlement to benefits and allowances, and these may be picked up in Post Offices and social security offices. With other financial problems, the bank manager may be of help.

SPIRITUAL NEEDS

Whatever the patient's beliefs, they should be respected. If he would like to talk to his minister, priest, rabbi or other religious adviser, a visit should be arranged. Make sure there is quiet and privacy during the visit and at any time when the patient would like to meditate or pray. Respect his wish to listen to or watch religious programmes on the radio or television.

You should be aware of two other possibilities. The patient may have no religious belief; in this case he should not be embarrassed or made to feel ashamed. Alternatively, your beliefs may not be the same as his; under no circumstances should you try to force your ideas upon him.

THE ROLE OF THE VOLUNTEER

In this country there has been a long tradition of voluntary effort and charitable work aimed at helping those in need. In recent years an increased emphasis has been placed on the work of the voluntary organizations.

THE VOLUNTARY ORGANIZATIONS

Today, the voluntary organizations play a vital part in assisting, and extending the work of, the statutory organizations. Volunteers are always available and ready to assist the professional – but will never replace her. It is in the home as a relative, a friend or a neighbour that most of the volunteer's caring is given.

As the needs of society change, so does the work of the volunteer. Patients are being discharged from hospital earlier, some to the care of the community nursing service but many to the care of their family. Many more are under-going minor investigations and operations as outpatients at hospitals rather than as inpatients. Patients with psychiatric disorders, some of whom have been in hospital for many years, are being re-habilitated back into the community, and here the companionship and friendship of an understanding volunteer can be invaluable to both the patient and the community psychiatric nurse. More and more elderly people are living on their own – these are people who often need help with daily routines when they are well, let alone when they are ill. Young and old with mental and physical handicaps and mothers with babies or young children may also need assistance.

The role of the volunteer has expanded greatly to meet all these needs. Much is an extension of "good neighbourliness"; some is more organized and linked to professional workers in the local community, such as in day centres and nurseries, residential homes and hospices. Wherever there is a need, volunteers are available.

Within some hospitals and Social Service Departments, the work of volunteers is coordinated by the Voluntary Service Organizer. This person has the task of identifying areas where volunteers can play a useful part, and recruiting and placing individuals where needed.

THE INDIVIDUAL VOLUNTEER

This book is primarily intended for members of the voluntary aid societies but will also be of use to those who choose or need to give nursing care at home. As a volunteer you hold a unique place in society. When you give nursing care you are accepted by the patient, his relatives and friends, and by the professional workers in the health care team. You are expected to have certain qualities: you should be energetic, imaginative, independent, able to work alone or as part of a team, always willing, always reliable and always self-controlled. You should use tact and discretion; you should demonstrate sincerity, sympathy, confidentiality and understanding. You also need special skills: you should be gentle and dextrous, observant, reassuring, resourceful, able to communicate easily with both patients and professionals, and able to give explicit instructions.

You should always look neat and tidy, as this can inspire confidence in the patient and his family. Your hair should be kept controlled and your nails short and clean. Shoes should be carefully chosen to provide support and to remain silent as you move around the sickroom. Many people smoke, but the smell of smoke on the breath may be nauseating to an ill person. You should also take care not to give offence from body odour. If you are careful about your own cleanliness and freshness, you are more likely to care about your patient's personal hygiene and appearance.

THE VOLUNTEER – PATIENT RELATIONSHIP

When someone is ill he becomes a patient. He will probably feel insecure and need the support of those around him. By going about your work in a quiet and confident manner you can quickly gain the respect and trust of the patient and his relatives. A good question to ask is: "How would I like to be cared for if I were ill?" If you can satisfy yourself then you will satisfy the patient. Remember that everyone has different likes and dislikes, so whenever possible involve the patient in the decisions that you make about his care.

Maintaining a good volunteer–patient relationship takes time as well as effort, but that is what nursing is: time, effort and skill in the service of others.

In the course of your work you may learn a great deal about a patient. It is essential to remember that information given to you by the patient or about the patient should only be discussed with the doctor, nurse or others professionally concerned with the care of the patient. What is said and done in the sickroom is not a subject for general comment or conversation outside it. Any instructions given by the doctor or professional nurse must be carried out punctually and carefully. There must be loyalty to the doctor and nurse at all times. If you observe these rules you will find that your relationship with those offering professional care is one of trust.

THE VOLUNTEER – PROFESSIONAL RELATIONSHIP

The professional members of the health team are responsible for the patient. As a volunteer, you are only there to assist them. It is essential that you recognize your own limitations and at no time try to exceed them. You should never make decisions or undertake treatment without prior consultation. You must recognize that you are privileged in being accepted as part of the caring team and you should be prepared in all things to put the patient first.

Reliability is a key element in your relations with doctors and professional nurses. If you undertake a ward duty you should expect to fulfil it on a regular basis – otherwise the ward sister cannot plan the use of your experience and may be irritated at the waste of her valuable time. You should be prepared to give a commitment to training and to keeping your skills up-to-date. If you do, you will find the professional nurse only too willing to help you gain the knowledge and the skill you need.

HOW TO USE THIS BOOK

Blue borders running round the edges of some pages in this book indicate those sections concerned with the care of babies and children. Blue boxes also appear on some other pages, indicating information relevant to those involved in child care.

Red boxes are used throughout the book to alert the reader to specific hazards that should be anticipated.

THE PATIENT'S SURROUNDINGS
HELPING THE PATIENT TO AVOID THE DANGERS OF THE ENVIRONMENT

Healthy people are usually able to choose their environment. If anything makes it uncomfortable or dangerous, they are free to make adjustments or move away. The person confined to bed is dependent upon those nursing him to see that his surroundings are safe.

As a volunteer, one of your tasks may be to provide a safe environment for the person in your care. When people are ill their movement is usually restricted. They may be confined to bed in their own home or in hospital. Their physical surroundings matter greatly and the bedroom and furniture should be selected with care. The general atmosphere in the room is also crucial. Family, friends, doctors and nurses all help to create it and their attitude largely determines whether or not the patient feels a burden. Always try to create a pleasant and cheerful atmosphere. Let the patient feel you have time to meet his every need. Be conscious of the privilege you have in serving the sick. Your forethought will give comfort to the patient as well as support to his family and friends.

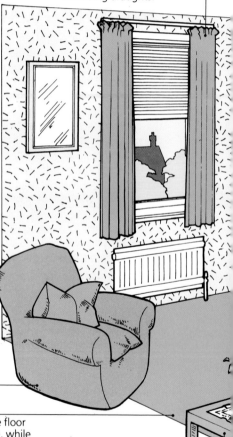

THE PATIENT'S ROOM

Curtains are most efficient for excluding draughts.

A comfortable armchair should provide good support for the patient's back when he is relaxing out of bed.

Carpet on the floor reduces noise, while also making it less likely that an unsteady patient will trip or slip. Avoid rugs.

A good-sized table becomes a surface on which to lay out equipment before treatment.

PLANNING THE PATIENT'S ROOM

The room in which the patient is nursed should be clean. The air can carry germs from one person to another and any dust stirred up can settle on food or a wound and so infect the patient. The room should also be free from unpleasant smells. Use an

A bedside cupboard provides the patient with a convenient surface for everything he needs to have within reach, as well as storage space. Provide a good bedside light and a handbell.

The ideal bed in which to nurse the patient is a single bed with access on three sides and a clear path between the bed and the door.

A commode of the type that doubles as an ordinary chair is useful for patients who cannot get as far as the bathroom.

A bed-tray is invaluable for the patient who has to have his meals in bed.

Two upright chairs are needed for visitors and for bedmaking.

aerosol to disperse the smells of food, bedpans and any other unpleasant odours – even flower water smells if it is not fresh. The sense of smell is intensified in sickness, so this is important.

The room should be comfortably warm and well ventilated. If it is too hot, the patient may sweat and become uncomfortable; if it is too cold, he may chill. Beware of draughts. In winter additional heating will probably be necessary. An open fire increases ventilation, but it should be well guarded so that when the patient is out of bed there is no danger of his dressing gown catching fire. Smoking in bed is also dangerous, particularly if the patient is elderly or drowsy. Always provide a large ashtray that will not spill easily and try to stay with the patient until he has finished smoking.

Most people prefer to stay in their own bedroom when they are ill. It may be more convenient for you to move a sick person downstairs or to a room nearer the bathroom, but do this only for his real well-being, not merely for your convenience. Whenever possible nurse the patient in a single bed with a firm but comfortable mattress. Try to leave plenty of space around the bed for ease of movement and the placement of any essential equipment.

If there is a pleasant garden or an interesting view, place the bed so that the patient can see out of the window. On the other hand, if the room can be overlooked there must be blinds or curtains that can be closed for privacy. These are also useful for controlling the light.

It is a good idea to leave everything the patient may need within easy reach of the bed, otherwise he may overbalance and fall when stretching for something or when getting out of bed to reach something. If a small hand bell is available, this is an added safety measure. A good bedside light is necessary for both patient and nurse, in addition to the main lighting.

With a confused patient, take care that nothing is left on his bedside table or within his reach that could cause him harm. Remove medicines, especially bottles of tablets, as he may repeat the dose forgetting what he has already taken.

Remove cigarettes and matches in case he sets the bed alight.

If the patient is able to use the bathroom you should ensure that the passageways are clear and light and that nothing has been left on the floor for him to trip over. Check that the bath water is not too hot and that there is a chair or stool in the bathroom.

Be sensitive to noise: to an ill person every sound seems magnified. Noise can cause headache and make the patient irritable. Carpeting on the floor and tablecloths on the bedside table and work surfaces will help to reduce noise and at the same time protect the furniture. You may need to turn down the radio and television or remove a ticking clock if it is disturbing him. Warn visitors to talk in a normal voice and not to shout: people often seem to think that because someone is ill he cannot hear.

Visitors, however welcome, can be exceedingly tiring for the sick or the old. If it seems necessary, try to restrict the number of visitors and the length of time they stay. This needs great tact and may tax your ingenuity if you are not to give offence.

Selecting furniture

If you are re-organizing a bedroom to make nursing easier, try to preserve the patient's feeling that it is still his room and his home. Individual needs will vary, but certain minimum requirements usually apply to all sickrooms:

You should have:

■ a firm table or locker for the patient within easy reach of the bed

■ an armchair for the patient to sit in when he is allowed out of bed

■ two chairs for bedmaking and for the use of visitors

■ a commode if one is necessary and available

■ a working surface for you: this should be protected by newspaper or plastic sheeting and covered with a clean paper towel

■ cupboard space, useful if there are any dressings or equipment that the community nursing sister or midwife might use

■ a clear pathway between the bed and the door so that neither you nor the patient stumbles into the furniture in the dark.

PLANNING A CHILD'S ROOM

The day of the formal nursery is past but, where possible, the new baby should have a room to himself, which in time can double as a playroom. The aim should be to provide a clean, airy room that is safe for its occupant. In the early months when the baby is confined to his cot there is little danger, but, once he begins to crawl, all sorts of hazards are to be found.

Parents usually re-decorate the room intended for the new baby; high gloss or washable paints and vinyl wallpapers are good choices as they are easily cleaned of grubby finger marks. A blackboard or an area of wall covered with formica gives the small child somewhere to draw and scribble as he wishes. The floor needs a covering as splinters from a wooden floor are danger-ous when the child is crawling; linoleum or lino tiles are safe and colourful and many of the new synthetic materials are both soft and warm to the knees. If rugs are used, they should be bright, washable and, above all, non-slip. Curtains too should be washable, and can be bright and colourful.

Ventilation is important and should be achieved without draughts. As the child grows you should take care to see that he cannot open a window himself nor fall out of one opened by you. Lighting should be adequate, but switches should be out of reach of small fingers and trailing flexes made inaccessible. Toddlers will push things into electric sockets: it is essential to put a plug into an empty socket even if it is unconnected to any equipment, or cover it with a specially designed safety socket cover, which are cheap to buy.

Heating is essential, especially for the newborn who may become severely chilled if the temperature drops at night. Central heating, oil-filled electric radiators or night storage heaters are probably the safest forms of heating but unfortunately are not always available. All fires should be adequately guarded. Gas fires may be dangerous if the flames blow out; ensure

regular servicing and adequate ventilation, as they can also cause condensation. Paraffin oil heaters should be avoided or used with great care as they account for innumerable deaths from fire each year among babies and children.

Selecting furniture

For the first few weeks of life a carry-cot is often the most useful and convenient item of baby's furniture, as it can be carried everywhere and the new baby put to sleep in it during the day as well as at night. If it has a waterproof hood and cover you will be able to take the baby out in the rain. If it comes with a stand and wheels it can double as a pram. Alternatively you may like to use a basket with handles. Although lighter and easier to carry than a carry-cot, such baskets are not waterproof and therefore not very practical for outdoor use.

As well as being convenient for you, the baby will also feel more comfortable and secure in the first weeks of life if he is in a small cot or cradle. By the time the baby is about six months old, however, a larger, more permanent cot will be needed: a drop-sided wooden one is probably the most hardwearing. The side-lowering mechanism should be sturdy but move easily. The cot bars should be no more than 8cm apart.

The cot mattress should be firm and encased in a waterproof material for easy cleaning – make sure the casing is plastic, not polythene. The mattress should fit the cot exactly so that there is no possibility of the baby becoming wedged in a gap between mattress and cot, and should be thick enough to keep the baby warm: if the mattress you have bought is a thin one, a folded blanket between the mattress and its waterproof cover will increase both the baby's warmth and his comfort. The sheets should be either flannelette or cotton. Flannelette sheets are warmer than cotton but take longer to dry. The bedclothes covering the baby should be light but warm; two cellular blankets, perhaps with an eiderdown, or a continental quilt and cover are commonly used alternatives.

A pillow is unnecessary and even dangerous for a baby under one year old: there is a chance that a small baby could bury his head in a pillow and suffocate.

How much other furniture you choose to put in the baby's room will depend on finance and personal taste, but, in the early days at least, you may possibly keep the baby bath and bathing equipment in the bedroom. There are two types of baby bath in common use: one is plastic and fits into a stand, the other fits over an ordinary bath. Both of these can be used until the baby is quite big. There should also be a low chair for you to sit on while you bath the baby. A trolley on wheels or a table is necessary for all the bathing equipment.

Cupboards are useful for clothing and for storing toys. As the child grows, a play-pen may be used: this allows freedom while restricting his environment to a safe one. Some kind of baby chair will also be needed; a low chair is safer than a high one. It should have a firm, broad base and safety straps to hold the baby in; its tray should be large and ideally should have rounded corners for easy cleaning.

THE BABY'S ROOM

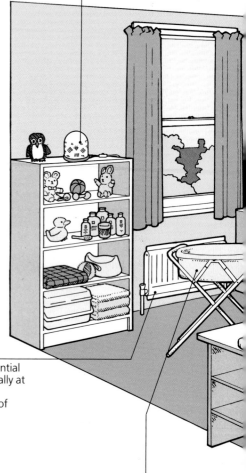

The child will need good lighting to play by as he gets older. Supplementary lighting, in the form of table lights and possibly a nightlight, will also become necessary.

Adequate heating is essential for the new baby, especially at night. Central heating is probably the safest type of heating to have.

Equipment for bathing the new baby may be best kept in the bedroom until he is big enough to be bathed in the ordinary bath. Some baby baths have their own stands, but many mothers prefer to bath the baby on a cupboard or work surface so that they can stand up.

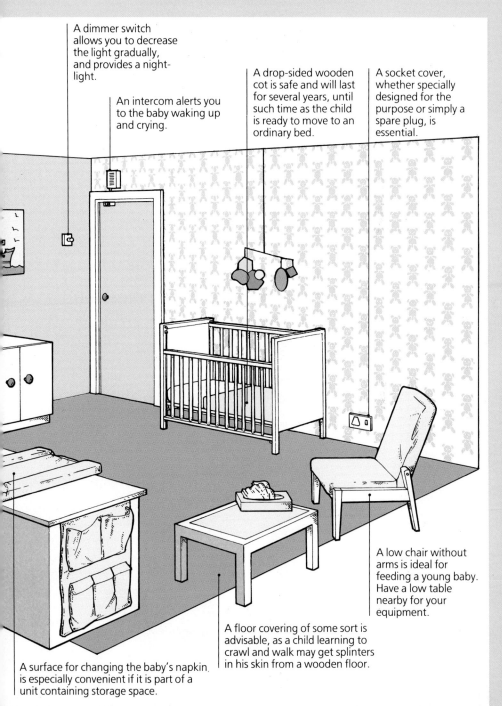

A dimmer switch allows you to decrease the light gradually, and provides a night-light.

An intercom alerts you to the baby waking up and crying.

A drop-sided wooden cot is safe and will last for several years, until such time as the child is ready to move to an ordinary bed.

A socket cover, whether specially designed for the purpose or simply a spare plug, is essential.

A low chair without arms is ideal for feeding a young baby. Have a low table nearby for your equipment.

A floor covering of some sort is advisable, as a child learning to crawl and walk may get splinters in his skin from a wooden floor.

A surface for changing the baby's napkin is especially convenient if it is part of a unit containing storage space.

COMFORT AND MOBILITY
HELPING THE PATIENT TO MOVE AND
MAINTAIN A COMFORTABLE POSITION

One of your most important tasks as a volunteer is to attend to the patient's comfort. Since much of the ill person's day is spent in and around the bed, you will need to make the bed neatly and regularly – whether or not he is allowed up.

If the patient is unable to move or if his movements are restricted, it is up to you to choose the most suitable position in bed for him: you should know how to lift and move him without causing any pain and without straining your back. Prolonged bedrest is

known to be harmful: a bedridden patient is likely to develop pressure sores (see page 29) and there is a risk of blood clotting in the leg veins (thrombosis). Because of this risk you should turn the patient regularly and help him to take gentle exercise. The community nursing sister will guide you in all these matters.

The patient who can get up and move around should be encouraged to do so; but do not forget that even the relatively mobile patient may need help.

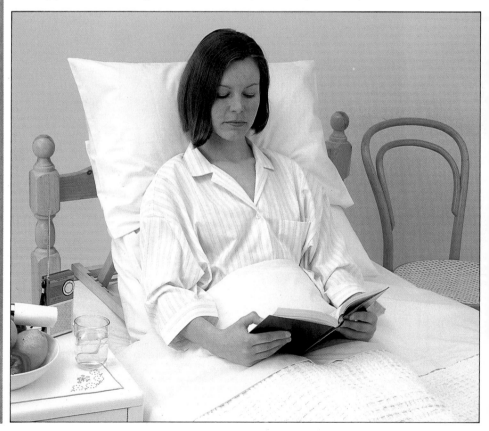

THE PATIENT IN BED

Most homes have low beds. These make nursing difficult, mainly because the risk of back strain for the helper is greater. Bed blocks can be placed under the bed legs to increase the height: they must be checked frequently as they may become unstable.

If the patient is being nursed in a double bed it is more difficult to care for him, especially if he cannot get out of bed. If there is a single bed available it might be worth trying to persuade him to move into that. However, having someone sharing the bed may alleviate distress and allay fears, particularly following a stroke or if a patient is handicapped; and any nursing disadvantage will probably be outweighed by the advantage of having another person at hand during the night.

Adjustable beds, which can be raised or lowered by a winding handle or hydraulic foot pedal, are expensive and usually found only in hospitals. The bed can be lowered when the patient is getting in or out and raised for bedmaking.

BEDMAKING

There are many different ways of making a bed, but certain rules apply at all times:
■ roll up your sleeves and remove watches and rings to prevent injury to the patient and damage to your personal possessions
■ strip the bed neatly (see below)
■ mitre corners (see page 26)
■ make sure there are enough bed-clothes at the top of the bed to fold back and still cover the patient when he lies down
■ loosen the bedclothes over the patient's feet so that he can move his toes freely.

To make a bed, you will need:
■ two sheets
■ an underblanket
■ two top blankets
■ an eiderdown in cold weather
■ as many pillows and pillow cases as the patient wants or his condition dictates
■ two chairs back to back.

If it is necessary to protect the mattress, you will also need a plastic sheet to go underneath the bottom sheet. Where a draw-sheet is used (see page 27), a piece of plastic sheeting can also be placed between that and the bottom sheet.

Stripping a bed
Two people should work together to strip a bed efficiently. Fold each layer of bedlinen neatly into three before removing it from the bed. Make sure the folded linen is placed tidily on two chairs and is not touching the floor, and that all the items are piled up in the order required to remake the bed.

Using a continental quilt
Continental quilts (duvets) are increasing in popularity: they are warm, light, mould themselves to the body and do not slip off the bed like an eiderdown. They come filled with down, a mixture of feather and down, or man-made fibres, and have washable covers. Quilts come in various sizes: use the largest available for the type of bed.

If a continental quilt suits the patient, bedmaking is greatly simplified. However, it is important to make the bed as often as you would normally. The patient needs the pleasure of returning to a freshly made bed in the same way as any other patient, and, although it is tempting to think that a quilt merely needs to be plumped up, the filling does tend to collect at the foot end, so the quilt will need a thorough shaking.

Change the bottom sheet in the usual way – often a fitted sheet is used (see page 27). The quilt replaces all the bedclothes on top of the patient. Shake the quilt so that its filling is evenly distributed and let it fall neatly on top of the pillows and bottom sheet. Avoid using a counterpane as it flattens the quilt and reduces the warmth created by the air trapped within the filling.

MAKING AN EMPTY BED

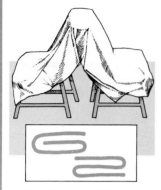

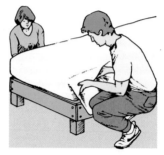

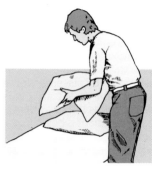

1 Fold the bedclothes neatly into three, following one of the two methods illustrated, and place them on two chairs at the end of the bed in the order you will need them. Work in pairs if you can.

2 Cover the mattress with the underblanket. Place the bottom sheet right side up with the crease centred down the middle of the bed. Tuck in along the head, then the foot of the bed, making mitred corners (see page 26). Pull the sheet taut before tucking in the sides.

3 Put pillows on the bed. Place the top sheet in position wrong side up, with the crease down the middle. Allow a 45cm turnover and half cover the pillow.

4 Tuck in the sheet at the foot of the bed. Make mitred corners and tuck in all along the sides. Repeat with each blanket. Place the counterpane on the bed with the sides hanging loose. Turn the top sheet down over the blankets and counterpane. Loosen the bedclothes at the end of the bed to enable the patient to move his or her feet without restrictions. NB: If using a duvet, shake it so the filling is evenly spread and lay it on the bottom sheet with no top sheet and no counterpane.

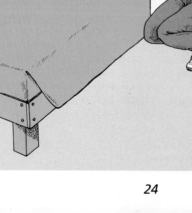

BEDMAKING WHEN THE PATIENT CANNOT GET UP

In these circumstances it is especially important that two people make the bed together. See that the room is warm and tell the patient what you are going to do before you start. Prepare a linen bag or bucket for any soiled linen. Put two chairs back to back at the foot of the bed.

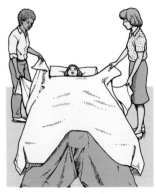

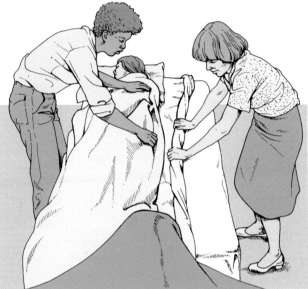

1 Loosen the bedclothes all around the mattress. Remove the counterpane by folding it in three and place it on the chairs. Remove all except one blanket in the same way. Slide out the top sheet, leaving the patient covered with the blanket, fold it into three and put it on the chairs. Remove all but one pillow, and place on the chairs.

2 Roll the patient to one side of the bed. Support her while your helper brushes out any crumbs, untucks the bottom layers of bedding and rolls them up to the patient's back. Your helper then straightens each layer in turn, pulling the underblanket and bottom sheet taut and tucking them in again.

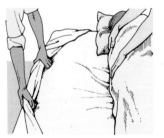

3 Roll the patient gently to the other side of the bed. Your helper now supports her while you repeat the process.

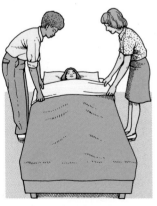

4 Sit the patient forward and replace the pillows. Unfold the top sheet over the blanket, then slide the blanket out from underneath, fold it and place on the chairs. Tuck in the sheet allowing 45cm turnover at the top. Replace the blankets one by one, tucking them in along the sides and more loosely at the foot of the bed. Replace the counterpane and turn down the sheet.

CHANGING THE BOTTOM SHEET

Roll the clean sheet lengthwise and place it on the chairs. With the patient rolled to one side of the bed and supported, your helper straightens the underblanket and plastic sheet as before, but leaves the soiled sheet rolled up close to the patient's back. She places the new sheet on the bed and tucks it in, then unrolls it to meet the soiled sheet. Roll the patient over both sheets and remove the soiled sheet. Straighten the underblanket and tuck in the new sheet.

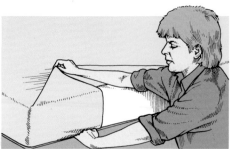

MAKING MITRED CORNERS

Pick up the edge of the sheet about 45cm from the top or bottom of the bed and pull it up. Make a triangle flat on the bed. Tuck in the edge that hangs down. Bring the triangular fold of sheet down over the top and let it hang. Pull it taut. Tuck it in.

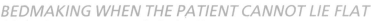

BEDMAKING WHEN THE PATIENT CANNOT LIE FLAT

If the patient cannot get up for bedmaking but cannot lie flat either – probably because she is breathless – remove the bedclothes (see page 25) but do not remove any pillows. Two of you should then lift the patient halfway down the bed. Your helper supports her while you make the top half of the bed. Remove the pillows and backrest, remove the drawsheet and place them on the chair. Brush out any crumbs. Roll the layers of bedclothes down to the patient's back, and straighten and tuck in the underblanket. Roll the sheet back and tuck in around the top half of the bed on your side. Support the patient while your helper does his side. Replace the drawsheet if used. Replace the backrest and pillows and lift the patient back up the bed. Repeat the process at the foot of the bed. Replace the top sheet and blankets as before.

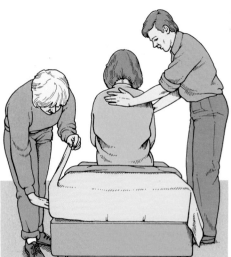
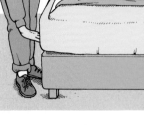

When changing the bottom sheet, roll the clean sheet up from its shorter edge. Follow the normal procedure, but this time working from the top downwards.

CHANGING A FITTED SHEET

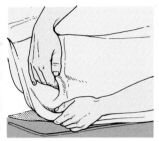

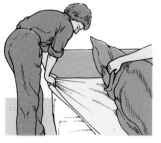

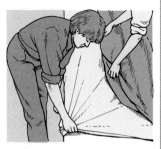

1 If the patient is in bed, proceed as opposite, rolling the sheet up lengthwise. Fit the top corner, then ease over the bottom corner.

2 Roll the patient over both sheets and remove the soiled one. Pull the clean sheet diagonally towards the top of the bed and ease over the corner.

3 Pull the sheet diagonally towards the bottom, bend up the mattress and ease the sheet over the last corner. Complete bed-making as before.

USING A DRAWSHEET

If the patient is in bed for more than a few days or is sweating a great deal, you may find a drawsheet useful. A drawsheet can be made from a rectangular piece of fabric about one metre wide and two metres long, or by folding a sheet in half lengthways. It is then placed on top of the bottom sheet under the patient's buttocks, and allows a clean cool area to be moved under the patient without there being any need to change the bottom sheet.

When you are making the bed, place the drawsheet on top of the bottom sheet. Tuck in one side, pull the sheet taut at the other side and tuck in the end first, then the slack. When the patient is uncomfortable and you want to adjust the drawsheet, untuck it at both ends. Pull a fresh area under the patient's buttocks, then tuck in at both sides again. The length of the drawsheet allows three or four clean areas to be pulled through before the sheet needs changing.

CHANGING A DRAWSHEET

1 Roll a clean drawsheet up from one short edge. Roll the patient on to his side and ask the helper to support him. Roll up the soiled drawsheet. Tuck in the clean drawsheet and unroll it until it meets the soiled one. Roll the patient over both sheets, remove the soiled one and gather the clean one in loose folds on the bed.

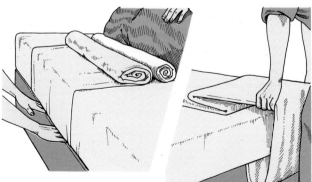

2 Tuck in the end. Pull out the folds and allow the slack to drop down. Pull taut and tuck in.

THE BABY'S COT

Making a cot is usually easier than making a bed, since only one person is needed and it is generally possible to lift the baby from the cot before you make it. Make sure he is warmly wrapped in a blanket first. Strip the bedlinen on to a chair.

A pillow is unnecessary and even dangerous for a baby under one year old.

To make a cot you will need:
- a mattress
- a waterproof cover (plastic, not polythene), unless the mattress has an integral one
- a cot bumper to fit around the top and sides of the cot, protecting the baby's head and upper body from draughts and accidental bumps
- a bottom sheet (fitted or other)
- a top sheet
- two cellular blankets
- a duvet in a cover instead of the last two items, if preferred.

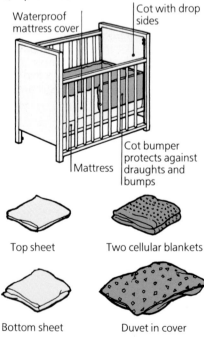

Waterproof mattress cover

Cot with drop sides

Cot bumper protects against draughts and bumps

Mattress

Top sheet

Two cellular blankets

Bottom sheet

Duvet in cover

WRAPPING THE NEW BABY

Very small babies often settle better if they are wrapped in one of the blankets or a flannelette sheet.

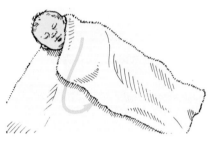

1 Bring one end of the blanket over his left shoulder and tuck it in behind him.

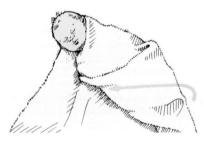

2 Hold the edge near the baby's left foot and bring it up to tuck in behind the baby again, folding the blanket on itself.

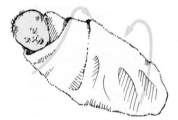

3 Bring the other end of the blanket over and tuck it behind the baby. Pull out the corner of excess fabric hanging down on the baby's right, bring it up diagonally and tuck it behind his back. Put him to sleep on his side.

PRESSURE AREAS

Whenever you sit or lie down you are compressing the skin and the underlying tissues between the bed or chair and your bones. But the compression is never so prolonged as to cause damage, because the pressure on the nerve endings in the skin causes healthy people to move frequently, even when asleep. However, if weakness, paralysis or unconsciousness makes movement impossible, if the patient is thin or very heavy, the pressure may be enough to cut off the blood supply to the underlying tissues. They then die and the skin ulcerates, and the ulcers are known as pressure sores. Common sites are: the back of the head; the shoulders; the elbows; the base of the spine; the buttocks; the sides of the hips; the knees; and the heels.

Some patients are more at risk than others. Those in good physical condition who are alert, fully mobile and continent are at far less risk of developing pressure sores than those in poor physical condition, who are confused, confined to bed, move with difficulty or who are incontinent. Other factors also contribute:

■ moisture next to the skin
■ wrinkles or crumbs in the bed
■ friction.

Preventing pressure sores
Improving the general health of the patient and the body's healing power with adequate protein and vitamin C (see pages 60–1) will help. Change the patient's position often –

about every two hours. Observe the skin regularly for redness, dryness or cracking, and inform the doctor if any of these signs are noticed. Keep the skin over the vulnerable area clean and dry, and be careful not to damage the skin when giving a bedpan. Make sure the bottom sheet is kept dry, taut and free from crumbs. Avoid friction: do not rub the area, and always lift, rather than drag, the patient up the bed.

If the patient is paralysed or incontinent, further measures can be taken. He may find that sitting on a sorbo ring or water cushion relieves pressure on the buttocks. Barrier cream may be used if he is incontinent. He may be helped by a ripple bed (alternating pressure mattress). This consists of a mattress of corrugated polythene, with an electric pump constantly inflating and deflating certain sections. An alternative is a water bed. This is a mattress filled with water that moves with the patient and so relieves pressure.

Treating pressure sores
If pressure sores occur, it becomes even more important to turn the patient regularly. Sores must be treated as surgical wounds. The doctor may remove dead tissue and pack the wound with gauze, either dry or soaked in a solution that aids healing. The pack allows the wound to heal from below upwards. The wound may also be treated with ultraviolet light, or other special measures may be followed.

Where pressure sores arise
The tinted areas indicate the areas most vulnerable to pressure sores in patients confined to bed. These areas are where the skin and underlying tissue is compressed between the bed and the bone. Pressure can be relieved in these specific areas with pillows, natural or artificial sheepskin, and sheepskin bootees for the feet.

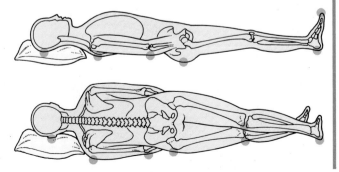

POSITIONS FOR BEDREST

There are five basic positions for bedrest, all of which can be modified to suit individual needs. The patient's condition may dictate the best position for him, but his comfort is a prime consideration.

The upright position (right)
The patient sits up with the back supported by several pillows, usually five, or by pillows and a backrest. Two of the pillows may be used to support his arms and a footrest used to prevent him from slipping down the bed.

The semi-recumbent position (right)
Three or four pillows support the patient's back. This is a comfortable position, allowing the patient to see around him and to eat and drink and converse without strain.

The recumbent position (below)
The patient lies flat on his back with one or two pillows. This can be restful and allows him to turn on his side.

The prone position (above)
The patient lies face down with pillows to support him. This position is used for soreness of the back or buttocks.

The recovery position (right)
This is used for the unconscious patient, who lies with his lower leg stretched out behind him, and his upper leg bent in front of him. His shoulders are tilted so that his lower arm is also behind him while his upper arm is bent in front. His head is turned to prevent the tongue blocking the airway. Note that there are no pillows – this is to prevent the patient inhaling his own vomit.

AIDS TO COMFORT IN BED

Backrests: When the patient is sitting up his back needs to be supported, and a backrest reduces the pillows required.
Footrests: It may be necessary to support the patient's feet to prevent him from slipping down the bed. In a long illness a foot support is also used to keep the foot at right angles to the leg.

Orthopaedic boards: Patients with back problems find it difficult to lie comfortably on a soft bed. The bed can be made rigid by one long board, or a series of boards, placed across the base under the mattress.

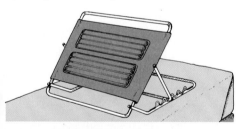

Adjustable backrest This standard type is widely available for use in the home.

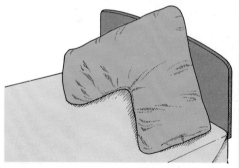

Triangular pillow This offers excellent support for sufferers from backache.

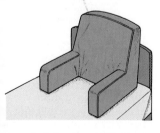

Armchair backrest This type is rigid and provides extra support for the arms.

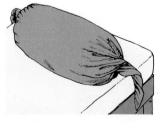

Footrest A soft footrest can either be a bolster or a pillow wrapped in a sheet.

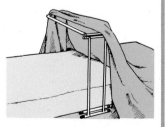

Bed cradle A cradle relieves the pressure of bedclothes on the feet and legs.

MOVING THE PATIENT

PROTECTING YOURSELF FROM INJURY

Moving a patient can cause you serious back injury if he is too heavy. Try to have a helper or mechanical aid available, and always follow these guidelines:
■ clear the floor space
■ keep your back straight: avoid arching it backwards or forwards
■ bend your knees, not your back

■ make your thigh muscles do the work
■ wear supporting shoes with low heels
■ always lift towards you, never away from you: this gives you better control.
  Encourage the patient to cooperate. Always *lift* him up the bed: never drag him. The following lifts are designed to protect you from injury.

SITTING THE PATIENT UP

You will want to sit the patient up for meals and as a change of position, but this is also the first step in lifting her or moving her from the bed to a chair (see page 35).

1 Fold the patient's arms across her waist. Place your inside knee on the bed level with her hip, and your outside foot on the floor in line with her waist. With your knee bent, put both hands well under her shoulder blades.

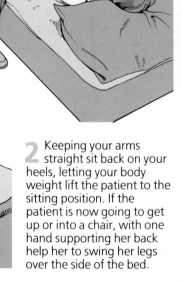

2 Keeping your arms straight sit back on your heels, letting your body weight lift the patient to the sitting position. If the patient is now going to get up or into a chair, with one hand supporting her back help her to swing her legs over the side of the bed.

LIFTING THE PATIENT UP A LOW BED BY YOURSELF

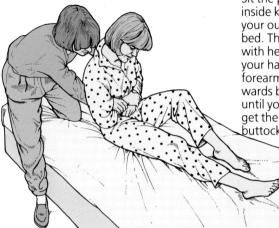

Sit the patient up (see opposite). Place your inside knee on the bed well behind her and your outside foot on the floor close to the bed. The patient should hold her right wrist with her left hand, and bend one knee. Slip your hands under her arms and grasp her forearms. Carry your body weight backwards by thrusting with your outside leg until you are sitting on your heel. If possible get the patient to straighten her knee. Her buttocks are now in line with your thigh.

DO NOT attempt to move a patient up a high bed without someone to help you (see page 34).

LIFTING THE PATIENT UP A LOW BED WITH A HELPER

This shoulder lift is suitable for two people working together. If you lift correctly, your backs should remain straight.

1 Sit the patient up and stand on either side of the bed. Place your inside leg on the bed level with the patient's hips. Sit back on your heel. Your outside leg should be on the floor the foot and knee in line with the patient's buttocks. Grasp your helper's forearm under the patient's thighs and press your shoulder into the patient's armpit. Rest your outside hand on the bed at the point to which you want to move the patient and have her arms resting on your backs.

2 On the count of "3" move the patient by thrusting with your legs and carrying your body forwards, pressing down with your outside arm. Maintain the pressure in the patient's armpit.

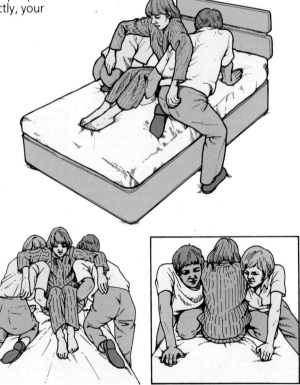

LIFTING THE PATIENT UP A LOW DOUBLE BED WITH A HELPER

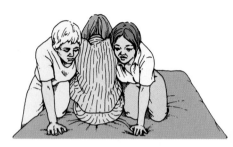

Move the patient to the side of the bed. With one helper proceeding as if you were lifting a patient up a low single bed (see page 33), the other should kneel on the bed, knees level with the patient's hips. Lift the patient by thrusting your body forwards, maintaining pressure in his armpits, and taking some weight on your outside arm.

LIFTING THE PATIENT UP A HIGH BED WITH A HELPER

DO NOT attempt to lift a patient up a high bed without someone to help you.

1 Stand at the side of the bed with your inside foot pointing at your helper and the other pointing at the bed head: make a 90° angle with your feet. Grasp your helper's forearm under the patient's thighs with your inside hand. Your inside shoulder should press into the patient's armpit and your outside hand should rest on the bed at the point to which you want to move the patient.

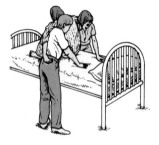

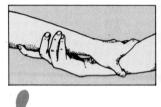

90°

2 On the count of "3" move the patient by straightening your knees, pressing down on the bed with your outside arm and shifting your weight to the leg nearest the top of the bed. Maintain the pressure in the patient's armpits. If you lift correctly, the patient should be raised and moved backwards.

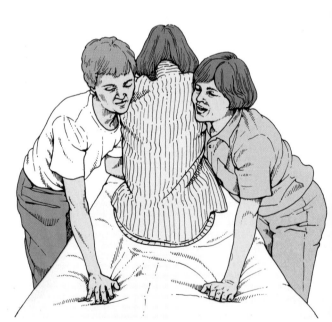

LIFTING THE PATIENT FROM A BED TO A CHAIR WITH A HELPER

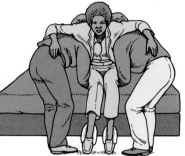

1 Place the chair in position. Sit the patient up with her legs over the side of the bed. Help her to put on her dressing gown and slippers. Grasp your helper's inside wrist under the patient's thighs. Press your shoulder into the patient's armpit, and place your outside hand flat on the bed. Your outside leg should be close to the bed with the foot pointing forwards, with your inside leg a little behind and the foot pointing inwards: your feet should form a 90° angle. With your back straight and your chin tucked in, bend at the hips and knees. Lift the patient by pressing into the patient's armpit with your shoulder while straightening your knees and pressing down on the bed.

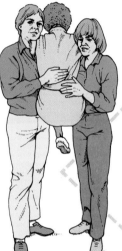

2 Support the patient's back with your outside hands as you walk towards the chair. When you reach it place your inside foot slightly in front of the chair, facing inwards, and your outside foot at the side of the chair, facing forwards: make a 90° angle with your feet. Lock your feet to prevent the chair moving. Place your outside hand on the arm of the chair. With your back straight and your knees and hips bent, lower the patient gently into the chair as your elbow bends.

HELPING THE PATIENT UP FROM A CHAIR

1 Stand slightly to one side of the patient and put one foot in front of hers to stop her sliding forwards. Make sure the chair cannot move. Bend your legs at the knee and place your hands under her armpits.

2 Keeping your back straight, straighten your legs and bring the patient into the standing position. Make sure she is steady before you move your feet and allow her to walk.

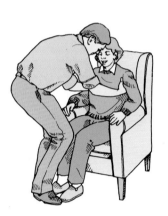
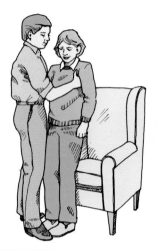

MOVING A PATIENT FROM A WHEELCHAIR TO A CHAIR (THE SWING LIFT)

1 Manoeuvre the wheelchair as near as possible to the chair or lavatory, and alongside it. Apply the brakes and remove the side piece nearest the chair or lavatory. Turn up the foot supports. Sit the patient with her knees at right angles and her feet on the floor. Stand in front of the patient.

Side piece removed

Footrest clear

2 Take a strong towel and fold it in half or thirds lengthwise. Grip the patient's knees between your own. Position the folded towel around her trunk under the armpits. Squat down to her height then, pivoting on your feet, pull her body up and swing it on to the lavatory or other chair.

If the patient can use her arms, ask her to help you by clasping you around the neck. Swing her up and out of the chair by clasping her upper arms or using the towel as a sling, as above.

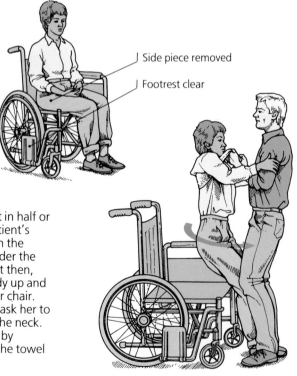

ENCOURAGING GREATER MOBILITY

Many patients recovering from a serious illness or an operation need help at first with walking and moving about. Elderly patients may also need help to a greater or lesser degree, as may the paralysed and handicapped. It is important to try and judge how much help the individual patient needs, and make it available to him without making him more dependent than necessary.

HELPING THE PATIENT TO WALK

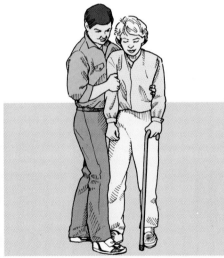

Patients recovering from a stroke that has temporarily paralysed one side of the body need special help to walk again. Stand at the patient's weaker side. Support her with one arm round her waist from behind and the other hand under her armpit from in front. Block her feet with your forward foot and prepare to use your knee to provide support for her weaker knee when she puts weight on it. Repeat to the patient:
- stick forward
- weak leg forward
- strong leg forward
until the rhythm is well established.

Helping the patient up stairs

Make sure the patient is not wearing anything loose that could trip him up. His shoes should provide support and have non-slip soles. You may need to take the patient's arm on the side opposite the handrail; or if he is extremely unsteady or the staircase exceptionally narrow, support him from behind by putting a hand under each armpit.

HELPING THE PATIENT INTO THE CAR

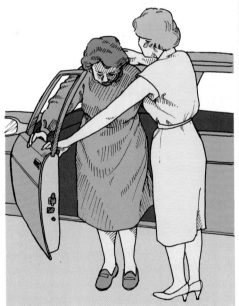

The patient who needs to visit the doctor or hospital for treatment may need help with getting in and out of the car. Open the car door wide and wind down the window. Holding the door open and protecting her head from the top of the door frame, get the patient to grasp the car door and turn round to sit down backwards. Lift her feet in if necessary. Reverse the procedure to help the patient out.

AIDS TO WALKING

If you are not actually helping the patient as he walks with an aid, keep an eye on him. Try to see that he finishes his walk in front of the chair he wants to sit in with the back of his legs touching it. Remove the walking aid, let him turn slightly towards his stronger side and encourage him to put his stronger hand on the chair arm or his hand on the seat before sitting down.

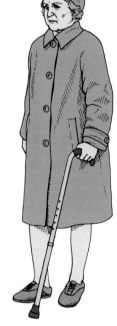

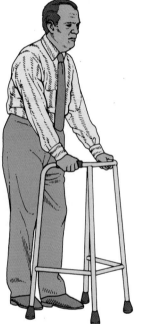

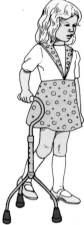

Portable canvas seat
A portable fold-up seat is useful for people who cannot stand for long. It is light and stable.

Tripod (left)
Tripods and quadrupeds are adjustable in height. They provide balanced support for those patients who need it.

Walking frame (above)
A Zimmer walking frame is ideal for someone who has to support some of his weight on his hands.

Stair lift (right)
In the case of a permanent disability or a condition such as breathlessness, it may be possible to install a stair lift on which the patient can stand or sit to ride up and down stairs. The social services will advise on this and in some areas will provide financial help.

Walking stick (above)
A stick with a rubber ferrule is ideal for a patient who only needs a little support.

THE PATIENT IN A WHEELCHAIR

As a volunteer or helper in the home, you may find that you have to care for a patient in a wheelchair. The help you give will depend on the type of patient involved. The disabled person confined permanently to a wheelchair will be very familiar with the way to use it and will probably instruct you about the specific help he needs, if any. But a temporarily incapacitated person of any age or a frail, elderly person may have to use a wheelchair for a while, yet may not be expert at handling it. These people are more likely to appreciate help.

Types of wheelchair
There are many different types of wheelchair, so before handling one you should examine it carefully. Note the position of the wheels and brakes, and establish whether the armrests and footrests are fixed or movable. In common use is the self-propelling type of wheelchair, with two large rear wheels. The outer rim fixed rigidly to each of these wheels makes it possible for the occupant of the chair to propel himself along. Chairs with four smaller

wheels are often lighter and easier to lift and push – but the occupant is dependent on someone to wheel him along. They often take up less space than the self-propelling types, and have pneumatic tyres, giving a more comfortable ride.

You may be involved in the care of a disabled patient who is moved from an ordinary to an electric wheelchair. Electric wheelchairs are usually operated from a lever on the armrest and run on batteries that can be recharged overnight from the mains. These chairs are expensive but offer the patient a large measure of independence. If you are helping a patient adjust to one, bear in mind that the controls are sensitive and require a degree of skill.

Helping the patient into a car
When you are helping the patient from a wheelchair to a car or vice versa, make sure that the brakes of both car and chair are fully on. Take note of how the patient wishes to be moved, and keep any clothing and blankets clear of the wheels. The swing lift (page 36) may be useful.

PUSHING A WHEELCHAIR DOWN A KERB

It is important not to startle or jar the patient in a wheelchair when negotiating a kerb. You will be successful as long as you take care to remain in complete control. With your foot on the chair's tipping lever hold the chair firmly and tip it back. Lower it slowly and gently down the kerb, making sure both back wheels touch the ground at the same time.

On the flat, do not push the chair so fast that she is frightened of being pushed out.

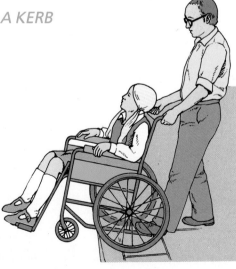

WASHING AND BATHING
HELPING THE PATIENT TO KEEP
HIS BODY CLEAN

The human body is covered with skin, which is a living tissue constantly renewed, the outer layers flaking away as they die. The skin contains sweat glands, sebaceous glands, hair, blood vessels and nerves. The sweat glands help to control body temperature: as the sweat evaporates it cools the skin. The sebaceous glands lubricate the skin and keep it supple. The hairs trap air: in man this is not very important, but it provides many animals with vital warmth. The blood vessels bring nourishment to the skin and carry away waste. The nerves provide information about temperature, pressure and touch.

The feverish patient sweats profusely and becomes hot, sticky, and uncomfortable. This is because the sweat glands in his skin are more active than usual. A regular part of your nursing care will be helping him to keep his body clean; in so doing you are removing stale sweat and allowing the glands to secrete freely. Try to assess how much help the patient needs, and offer any useful aids. Be prepared to wash, shave and bath him, and help care for his mouth, nails, hair and eyes if this proves necessary.

Cross-section of the skin

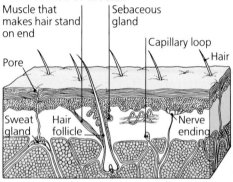

Muscle that makes hair stand on end — Sebaceous gland — Capillary loop — Hair — Pore — Sweat gland — Hair follicle — Nerve ending

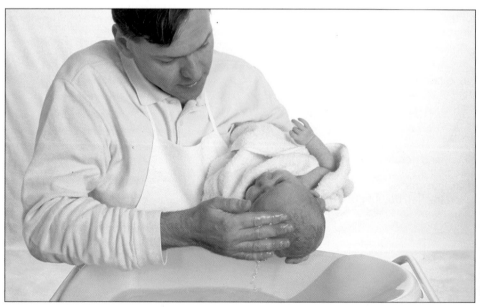

BATHING IN THE BATHROOM

If the patient is mobile enough, he can bath in the bathroom, perhaps with the help of bathing aids. If the patient is confined to bed or very inactive, he can be bathed in bed. This is known as a bed or blanket bath and includes caring for the nails, eyes, hair, mouth and teeth (see pages 44–48).

A daily bath is ideal – though it is as well to check how often the patient would normally bath. Some elderly patients are nervous of bathing, and if so a good wash down can be just as adequate.

Bathing provides you with an important opportunity to observe the patient carefully; if you notice any changes in the colour and appearance of the skin, report them immediately.

Make sure that the bathroom is warm. Gather together soap, flannels, towels, talcum powder and any clean clothes that may be wanted. Run the cold water in first, then run in the hot and mix thoroughly. Tell the patient that his bath is ready and, if necessary, help him to the bathroom. You may need to offer help with getting into and out of the bath (see pages 42–3).

Some patients may need help with washing and drying, others will be well enough to be left alone. A patient should not lock the door, however, and should have a bell within reach. Never leave a child or a confused person alone in the bathroom.

After the patient has left, clean the bath and leave the room tidy.

AIDS TO BATHING

A handrail or a bath seat may make it possible for a frail or elderly person to bath alone. If you are caring for a heavy or disabled patient, you might be able to borrow a hoist, a device used to lift people into the bath. The correct type must be recommended by a therapist, who will also teach you how to operate it.

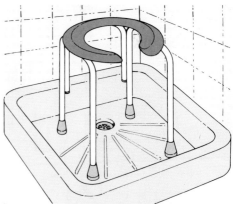

Shower seat (above)
The elderly, disabled, or those who find it hard to sit down in the bath may prefer a shower, with a seat.

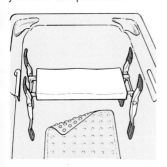

Bath seat (above)
Bath seats help patients who find it hard to get down to the bottom of the bath. There are many different types available. A mat held firm by suction pads is also very useful.

Handrail (left)
There are many different sorts of handrail. Some can turn out to be dangerous, so get expert advice before choosing one.

GETTING IN AND OUT OF THE SHOWER AND BATH

Helping a patient into the shower or bath is not easy, and you should follow the guidelines for moving a patient on page 32, particularly when helping him into or out of the bath: avoid injury to yourself by keeping your back straight, bending your knees, and taking the weight on your legs and arms.

Depending on the amount of help the patient requires in the bath, follow one of the two methods illustrated here. A non-slip mat (see page 41) in the bath will help.

To help a patient out of the bath, follow the procedure in reverse. If the patient finds it hard to get up, drain the water, cover him with a warm towel and step into the bath yourself. Bend your knees, place your hands under his armpits, straighten your legs and lift him upright.

HELPING THE PATIENT INTO THE SHOWER

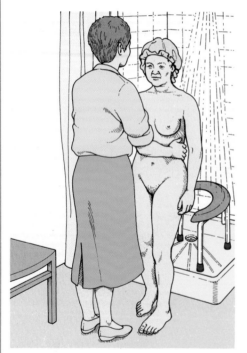
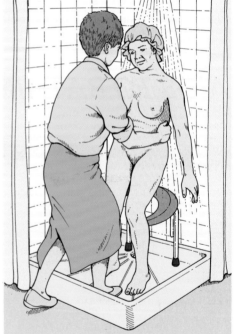

1 Position a chair near the shower. Place the shower seat in the correct position in the shower. Turn the water on and adjust to the right temperature, making sure it is not too hot. Help the patient to remove her nightdress and seat her on the chair. Help her to stand up, make sure she is steady, then help her to walk to the shower. She should stand with her back towards it.

2 With your knees bent and your back straight, gently lower the patient on to the shower seat. Offer her any help she needs as she washes. Do not leave the room. When she has finished, turn the water off, then help her out on to the chair.

HELPING THE PATIENT WHO NEEDS A MODERATE AMOUNT OF HELP (THE ELDERLY) INTO THE BATH

1 Stand behind the patient and get him to grasp his wrist with his other hand. Slip your hands under his armpits and firmly grasp his forearms in front of his waist.

2 Let the patient put both feet into the bath. Keeping your back straight and making your leg muscles do the work, bend your knees and lower him on to a bath seat or the floor of the bath.

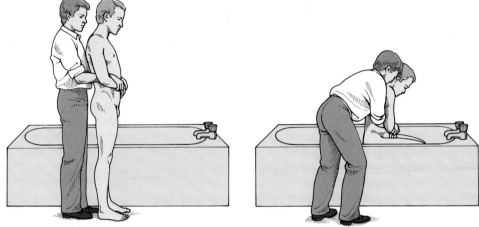

HELPING THE PATIENT WHO REQUIRES A LITTLE HELP (THE CONVALESCENT) INTO THE BATH

1 Stand facing the patient sideways on to the bath and place your hands under his arms. Help him lift his inner leg into the bath.

2 To straighten up, the patient pushes on your shoulders, swings his other leg in and grasps the sides of the bath. With your hands under his armpits, lower him gradually into the bath.

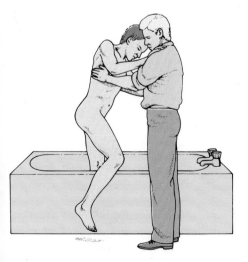

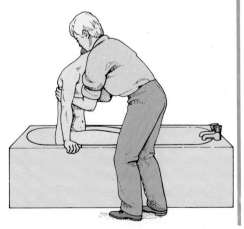

GIVING A BED BATH

A bed bath will be necessary if the patient is too ill or immobile to make the journey to the bathroom.

Make sure that the bedroom is warm and that the windows are closed.

You will need:
■ a bowl of hot water
■ soap
■ two towels
■ a face flannel
■ a body flannel
■ talcum powder
■ toilet water
■ a deodorant
■ a change of clothing
■ a brush and comb.

Remove the top bedclothes, but leave the patient covered with a blanket. Help to take off pyjamas or nightdress. Place a towel underneath each part as you wash it to protect the bed. First wash, rinse and dry the face, neck and ears; if the patient is well enough he may do this for himself.

Wash, rinse and dry one arm from the armpit to the fingers, then repeat with the other. Let the patient rinse his hands in the bowl of water. Wash and dry the patient's chest and abdomen. Powder under his arms or use a deodorant if appropriate. Wash and dry each leg in turn: when possible flex his knee and rinse each foot in the bowl after washing, as this is very refreshing. Many patients can wash the groin and genital area for themselves, if you hold the blanket out of their way. Very ill or unconscious patients will not be able to, and you will need to wash this area for them: you may find it easier with the patient lying on his side. Roll him on to his side to wash his back as well.

As you wash the patient, keep him covered as much as possible. Change the water whenever it cools and after the genital area has been washed. When you have finished, help the patient to put on clean nightwear. (If possible, keep separate clothing for night-time.)

After bathing the patient, help him to clean his teeth, brush his hair, and to shave (see opposite). Make-up may boost the morale of a female patient. Remake the bed, clear the room and open a window.

Washing the patient's back
Roll the patient on to his side so that his back can be washed. If you are alone turn him towards you to minimize the risk of him falling out of bed.

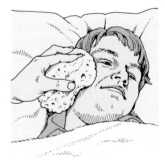

Washing the patient's face
If the patient wants you to wash his face for him, ask him first if he likes soap.

WASHING

Bear in mind that, as well as bathing, the patient needs to wash at other times. Washing his hands and face often refreshes an ill person and makes him feel more comfortable. Make a point of offering the patient confined to bed a face flannel and a bowl of warm water several times a day. He should also wash his hands after using a bedpan or commode, or going to the lavatory. Offer the female patient hand lotion.

SHAVING

A man who shaves regularly will find it both uncomfortable and embarrassing when stubble grows. If he is unable to shave himself, then you must do it for him.

Assess the patient's condition and judge how much help he needs. Ask him what kind of razor he normally uses – switching from an electric to a safety razor will cause him discomfort for several days. Also find out in which direction he shaves: the bristles grow according to the direction of shaving, and going against the normal lay causes pulling and tenderness. Protect him and the bed with towels.

Shaving with a safety razor
Lather the chin, rubbing soap well in: this softens the beard and makes the shave more comfortable. Rinse his face, then re-lather and shave him in the direction he has indicated. Take long, firm strokes and rinse the razor frequently. When you have finished, rinse the patient's face and dry it thoroughly. Use after-shave lotion if he would like it. Remove the towel, clear away and clean the razor.

Shaving with an electric razor
If the patient uses an electric razor, check that it is clean. Shave the patient's face in the correct direction before you wash it. Allow the razor to cut the stubble, never scrub across the face. Pre-electric or after-shave lotions may be used if the patient likes them. Remove the towel, clear away and clean the razor.

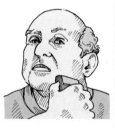

Using a safety razor
Shave in long, firm strokes in the direction preferred by the patient, rinsing the razor frequently.

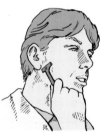

Using an electric razor
Shave in the direction preferred by the patient *before* washing his face.

CARING FOR THE NAILS

You will have the opportunity to notice if the patient's nails need attention while you are bathing him. You may find you have to use a nail brush to keep his nails clean, and you should also remember to cut the nails regularly; fingernails should be cut or filed to the shape of the finger, while toenails should be cut straight across. The female patient may enjoy a manicure and some nail varnish if you have time.

It is not uncommon for elderly people to have very hard and horny nails. The help of a chiropodist is invaluable in these cases: an elderly person can be housebound because of his toenails and the chiropodist can, quite literally, put him on his feet again. But although health authorities are obliged to provide a chiropody service, it is often inadequate. The voluntary organizations may also provide foot care.

CARING FOR THE EYES

In normal health the eyes are kept moist and clean by a film of fluid that flows across the eyeball and drains into the nose. In illness, however, the eyes may become dry, sore and occasionally infected. It may be hard for the patient to open them properly, and you will need to bathe the eyes to clean them.

You will need:
■ a tray
■ cotton wool swabs
■ a bowl of clean water or a saline solution (one 5ml spoonful of salt to 600ml of previously boiled water)
■ a paper towel or square of kitchen paper
■ a paper bag for used swabs
■ eye drops if prescribed (see pages 78–9).
Help the patient into a comfortable position and tell him what you are going to do. If he can lie flat, you can stand behind his head, the ideal position from which to treat the eyes. If this is not possible see that the patient's head is back and his shoulders supported. Wash your hands. Arrange the towel under his face. Dip a swab into the water or saline solution, squeeze it gently, and swab the eye from the nose outwards. Discard the swab. Repeat the procedure until both eyes are clean. Dry the surrounding skin with clean, dry swabs. Use each swab *once only*, to prevent cross-infection.

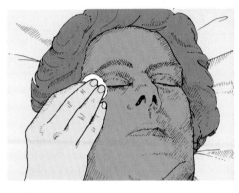

Bathing infected eyes
Swab the affected eye from the nose outwards. Use each swab once only.

CARING FOR THE MOUTH

After each meal, minute particles of food are left behind in the mouth. These particles begin to decompose and harmful bacteria flourish and multiply. As well as leaving an unpleasant taste and feeling in the mouth, these bacteria can cause tooth decay or mouth infections.

It is therefore essential to keep the mouth clean. The healthy person will clean his teeth regularly to remove plaque and debris, but patients confined to bed are unable to care for their mouths without assistance. In many cases, all you need do is provide them with the means to clean their teeth at regular intervals. As well as toothbrush and toothpaste, give the patient a glass of water and a bowl to spit into. Check whether he prefers warm or cold water.

Unless the doctor forbids it, leave a jug of water within the patient's reach and encourage him to drink. Mouthwashes are refreshing for a short period: offer sharp-tasting fruit juices sometimes as an alternative to brand-name antiseptic varieties. Juice is less monotonous than brand-name mouthwashes, and is preferable for children or confused patients as they will come to no harm if they accidentally swallow it. The sharp flavour of the juices encourages the glands to produce saliva, which is antiseptic and cleans the mouth. Chewing gum and small pieces of fruit – such as fresh pineapple – also cause saliva to flow.

In some cases the patient may be too ill or weak to attend to his own mouth and you must do it for him. All ill patients should have their mouths cleaned several times a day, both before and after meals. Done frequently, cleaning the mouth takes only a short time, but if the mouth is neglected, cleaning it becomes a difficult task for you and an ordeal for the patient. Research has

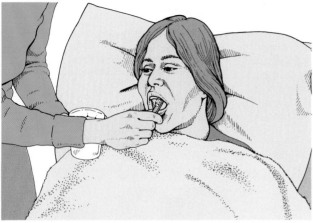

Cleaning the patient's mouth
Clean the mouth from the top downwards: clean the gums and all surfaces of the teeth using an up and down and side to side movement. Brushing is the only effective way of removing plaque and debris.

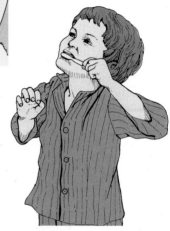

shown that the most satisfactory way is with a child's soft toothbrush and toothpaste, preferably one containing chlorhexidine. If the mouth is encrusted with mucus, however, substitute a solution of bicarbonate of soda for the toothpaste.

You will need:
- a tray
- a child's soft toothbrush
- toothpaste, preferably with chlorhexidine, or a small container holding bicarbonate of soda solution (one 5ml spoonful of powder to 600ml of water)
- a small container of water or mouthwash and a bowl to rinse into
- cream, lip salve or Vaseline for dry lips.

  Help the patient into a comfortable position and tell him what you are going to do. Wash your hands, before tucking the towel under the patient's chin. Using toothbrush and toothpaste, or the bicarbonate of soda solution, clean all the surfaces of the mouth. Help the patient to rinse with water or mouthwash. Apply the lip salve, if the lips are dry.

Cleaning the child's teeth
As soon as a child is old enough, get him into the habit of cleaning his teeth twice a day. Also try to restrict his intake of sticky, sweet foods.

Denture care
Get the patient to remove his dentures and place them in a container. Take them to the bathroom and brush them with denture cleaner or toothpaste under cold running water. If the dentures are stained, soak them in a special solution. Rinse thoroughly before returning them to the patient.

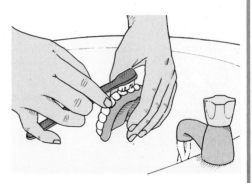

Cleaning dentures
Brush dentures thoroughly under cold running water to remove particles of food. Use denture cream or toothpaste. Clean them in a stain-removing solution as often as necessary.

CARING FOR THE HAIR

Brush and comb the patient's hair at least twice a day, and arrange it in a style that is easy to manage and pleases the patient.

Anyone who has been ill for a long period will probably need his hair washed. A local hairdresser may be willing to visit the home, but they will almost certainly want the patient to sit at a handbasin.

If you need to wash the patient's hair in bed, first help the patient into a suitable position. This could be lying back with a bowl under her head, or sitting up in bed and leaning over a bowl on a bed-table. Protect the bed and surrounding floor by covering both patient and bed with a liberal supply of waterproof material and the floor with plastic sheeting or newspaper. Find out what shampoo and conditioner the patient prefers. Wash the hair thoroughly and rinse it well in clean water. Use a hair dryer if there is one available, otherwise rub the hair dry with warm towels. Finish by brushing and combing it so that it looks attractive.

Washing the hair in bed
The patient can lie back on the bed with a bowl under her head and her shoulders raised on pillows covered with plastic sheeting.

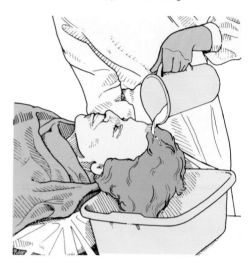

EXAMINING AN INFESTED HEAD

Lice infestation can affect both clean and dirty heads of hair, whether standards of cleanliness are high or not. Lice multiply quickly by laying eggs, which are called nits and stick to strands of hair.

Lice spread in crowded conditions, especially amongst schoolchildren. If an infested head is found, ask the other members of the family for permission to examine their heads. Once you have treated the condition, examine the hair regularly to check that there is no recurrence.

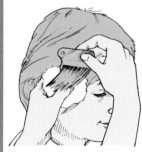

1 Protect the patient's shoulders. Dip a fine tooth-comb into disinfectant solution. With a swab in one hand, comb the hair from roots to tips.

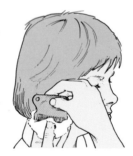

2 Wipe the comb on the swab after each stroke. Examine it for lice and inspect the hair for nits. Scurf will brush out but nits stick firmly to hairs.

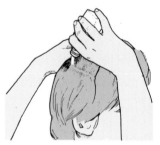

3 If lice are found, apply a chemical compound such as malathion or carbaryl. Follow the manufacturer's instructions, and protect the eyes.

BATHING THE BABY

It is unnecessary, particularly in very cold weather, to bath a baby every day: "topping and tailing" cleans the important areas. Wash and dry the face gently using cotton wool balls. Clean the napkin area with soap and water or baby lotion.

To give the baby a proper bath, make sure first that the room is warm and the windows closed.

You will need, close at hand:
■ baby bath liquid, or baby soap and baby shampoo
■ baby lotion
■ cotton wool swabs
■ a soft flannel or a sponge
■ a large soft towel
■ a change of clothing
■ a clean disposable napkin, or a clean terry napkin, liner, plastic pants and safety pins
■ a bucket for soiled clothes
■ a paper bag for soiled swabs.

Fill the bath, putting the cold water in first, then adding hot until the water feels warm to your elbow. Add the bathing liquid.

BATHING THE NEW BABY

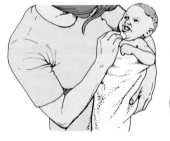

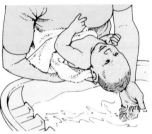

1 Undress the baby apart from his napkin and wrap him in a towel on your lap. Clean his face with cotton wool balls or a soft flannel and dry it carefully.

2 Hold him along your arm, his head towards the bath and on your hand. Rinse his hair and pat dry. Remove napkin and clean the buttocks.

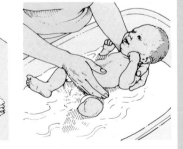

3 If using baby soap, lather your hands and soap the baby. Support the baby's head and shoulders on one hand and forearm, with your other hand underneath his bottom and holding the thigh furthest from you. Lift him into the bath. Keep his head and neck well supported. Smile and talk to him, making bathtime fun.

4 Use your free hand to wash and rinse him. Lift him out carefully using the same grip. Wrap him in the towel and pat him dry. Check his creases are dry.

49

CLOTHING
HELPING THE PATIENT TO DRESS AND UNDRESS AND TO SELECT CLOTHING

Choice of clothing is a very personal thing and both patients and their relatives will probably have fixed ideas about what they like and dislike. Cultural or religious traditions may also determine the clothes they wear. However, if illness or disability makes it necessary to adapt clothing for a specific need, most people appreciate help.

This means that, as well as being able to help dress and undress the patient and offering dressing aids to make it easier for him to dress and undress himself, you should also find out what special clothing is available for his particular disability, and what adaptations you can make to his existing clothing. You may find you have to learn to help someone with a garment that is unfamiliar to you, such as a sari, for example. Remember that, in helping the patient to select the right clothing for his condition, tact is just as important as the choice itself. Be careful not to cause embarrassment by suggesting items which are out of the patient's price range, for example, or which make patients feel more conscious of their particular problem.

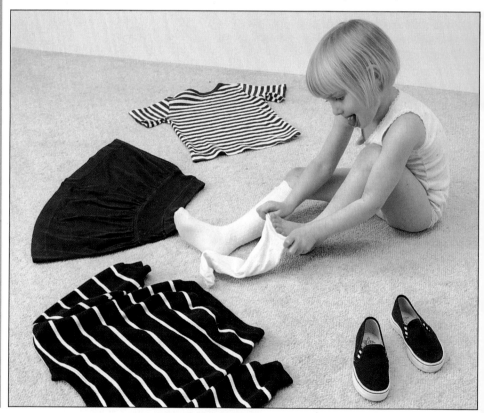

DRESSING AND UNDRESSING

It is wise to encourage the patient to do as much for himself as he can. This may make dressing and undressing lengthy processes if he is blind, stiff, weak from old age, arthritic, has lost a limb or is paralysed as the result of an injury or stroke. But they are important routines in the patient's day: every achievement is a step towards independence. Allow the patient plenty of time for dressing and undressing and provide any dressing aids appropriate to his disability. Encourage him to rest at intervals.

SLEEVES OVER ARMS

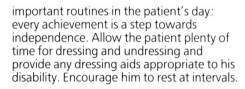

If one arm is injured or paralysed, deal with it first. Slip your hand up through the sleeve from the cuff and grasp the patient's hand. Slide the sleeve of the garment along her arm and round her back, pulling the garment not the patient.

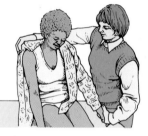

TROUSERS OVER LEGS

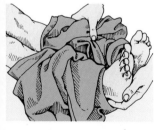

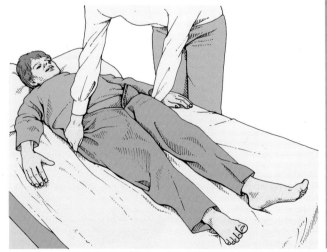

With the patient laying on the bed, slide the trousers over one foot, then the other. Pull them up. Help the patient to lift his buttocks off the bed while you ease the trousers up to the waist. Tuck in the shirt and fasten them.

Right: If the patient is lying down, slip her arms into the garment first, then ease the neck opening over her head.

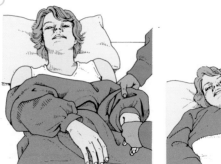

Far right: If the patient's arms both function, slip the garment over her head first, then help her arms into the sleeves.

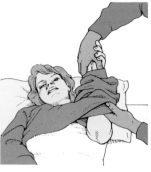

AIDS TO DRESSING

Tasks that most people take for granted become impossible when a person is weak or arthritic. With the help of a few simple aids, however, such a person may find it possible to continue dressing himself and so retain his dignity.

Dressing stick (right)
A dressing stick can be made from an old coat-hanger and a rubber thimble. The V-shaped notch pulls straps over the shoulder; the rubber thimble clings to fabrics.

Shoe horn (below)
This long-handled shoe horn helps people who cannot bend down easily.

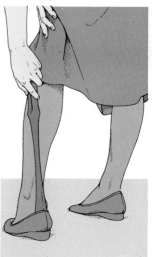

Stocking aid (above)
A stocking aid has a plastic frame over which the stocking is slipped. The toes can then be pushed in and the stocking and frame pulled up by means of the handle.

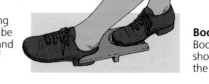

Boot jack (left)
Boot levers or boot jacks enable shoes to be removed without the patient bending down.

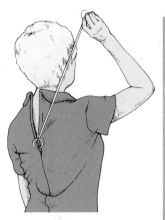

Lazy tongs (above)
Lazy tongs have a mechanism at the top of the handle which operates the jaws at the bottom.

Extend-a-hand (right)
An extend-a-hand performs the same function as lazy tongs but is of adjustable length.

Zip aid (above)
Zips can be pulled up more easily by either a hook on a cord or a piece of string threaded through the zipper.

SELECTING CLOTHING

Before selecting clothing, consider any specific problems the patient may have. People who are incontinent, handicapped, confined to a wheelchair, partially sighted or who have arthritic hands all need careful individual consideration. With a little ingenuity, many ordinary items of clothing can be adapted to individual needs.

Once you have taken the particular circumstances into account, the style of clothing selected will also depend on the weather and the kind of activity the patient is likely to undertake. Clothes should preferably all be light, easily washed and dried and require little or no ironing. Flame-resistant fabrics are best wherever possible, especially for the nightwear of children and incapacitated people. If the fabric is man-made, it should be 100 per cent polyester, which tends to melt in contact with fire; never choose acrylic, which will flare up.

The type and style of clothing chosen will depend very much on specific needs but it must look attractive and fit well to boost morale. Shoes should be comfortable and give support. The slip-on shoe is the easiest to manage but you can buy elastic laces if the patient prefers lace-up shoes. Slippers should be discouraged, especially for a patient who has had a stroke.

If the patient's clothing needs protecting at mealtimes, a plastic apron or a small make-up cape may do the job. For a female patient who is more severely incapacitated, a dress with a protective front may be useful – the front can be added at mealtimes and removed when not required.

There are many modifications to clothing that will help patients whose hands are weak or arthritic. Front fastenings and wrap-over skirts make dressing easier for female patients. Conventional fastenings can be replaced with Velcro. Special braces, known as Edgware braces, can make it easier for the patient with the use of only one arm to take his trousers on and off: these braces are attached to the middle of the back of the trousers and worn round the neck like a school satchel. To put the trousers on, the patient sits down to pull them up as far as he can and to lift the braces over his head. When he stands up, the braces pull the trousers up over his buttocks, with the help of his hand.

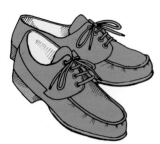

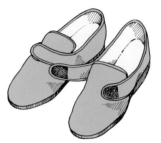

Non-tying tie
Ties can be bought ready-tied and attached with a clip or with Velcro. They look just like normal ties.

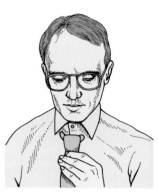

Elastic laces
A lace-up shoe provides some support, and elastic laces help people who can't tie knots.

Velcro shoe fastenings
Patients who can't manage fastenings but don't like slip-on shoes may like shoes fastened with Velcro.

Wrap-over skirt
A wrap-over skirt with its fastening at the front is comparatively easy for a patient with weak or arthritic hands to deal with.

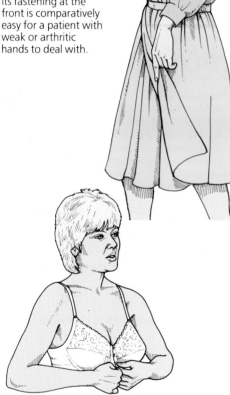

"Hold-up" stockings
Suspenders can be avoided by choosing stockings with a welt at the top that is designed to stop them falling down, but without restricting the circulation in the legs.

Single-leg tights
The advantages of both tights and stockings are combined in single-leg tights. These eliminate the need for suspenders, and allow more air to circulate than tights.

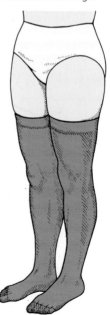

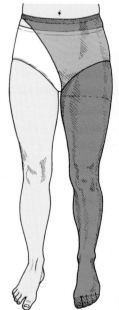

Front-fastening brassiere
This simplifies a daily task that can seem extremely difficult to those with weak or arthritic hands.

Brassieres with front fastenings may help the arthritic or paralysed patient; patients could also fasten a back fastening in front and rotate it to the back. After the removal of a breast (mastectomy), a "criss cross" bra, or a style supplied by the National Health Service, is the most suitable.

Women with arthritic hands may find tights easier to cope with than stockings and suspenders. Tights do exclude the air and some people find them uncomfortable; they also seem to increase the likelihood of vaginal infections. Both problems can be avoided by buying single-leg tights, tights with cotton gussets or tights with no gusset, all of which allow air to circulate more freely. Garters are not a good idea, as they often impede circulation. If the patient finds pulling pants up and down difficult, there is a special crotch vent knicker available which she may find useful.

Clothing for the incontinent

Incontinence brings many problems, but garments that open easily, have wrap-over backs or conceal drainage bags alleviate some of them.

For those female patients whose problem is the inability to wait rather than true incontinence, French knickers and single-leg tights may prove easier to manage than many other underclothes.

Garments with wrap-over backs have two flaps that can be moved from under the buttocks when the patient is sitting or lying, so avoiding soiling. Nightdresses, dressing gowns, dresses and slips are available with wrap-over backs, in pleasant and easily-washed fabrics. These clothes give comfort and security to the incontinent, and are labour-saving for those providing care; but they do not provide an excuse for not using the lavatory as often as is necessary.

For men, Velcro fastenings and elastic waist-bands make trousers easier to cope with. Suits can be adapted for easy movement and flies enlarged to accommodate urinals and other appliances. Trousers can be modified to incorporate a flap in the back; a long open-back shirt is available; and for those wearing pyjamas for long periods the U-shaped crotch and raglan sleeve make movement easier.

Many other normal garments can be adapted: long zips or Velcro fastenings can be added; dresses can open right down the front; a skirt may be opened down both sides and the front panel secured around the waist with tapes, allowing the back panel to be pulled down easily. Some Women's Royal Voluntary Service centres and other organizations may give help with alterations. The community nursing sister, social worker for the disabled or Citizens' Advice Bureau will be able to provide you with information about where special clothing may be selected and bought.

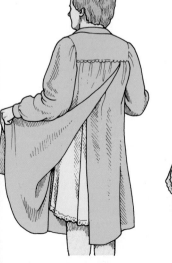
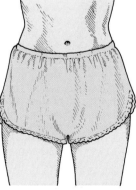

French knickers (left)
Commonly available, French knickers have the advantage of a wide leg opening. They are useful if the patient is often in a hurry to use the lavatory.

Wrap-over dress (far left)
A dress with a wrap-over back looks perfectly normal when the patient is standing or walking about. When she is sitting or lying down, the two flaps at the back can be opened and pushed back so that she is in no danger of soiling them.

DRESSING THE NEW BABY

In the first months of life most babies do not like to be naked: without a wrapping of some sort they feel insecure (see page 28). Their intense dislike of being undressed can make dressing and undressing an ordeal for both you and the baby. Because of this you should proceed with as little fuss as possible, remembering to pull the clothes rather than the baby's limbs. If the baby seems very unhappy when he is naked, however securely you are holding him, try leaving a clean folded napkin on his tummy while you are removing the rest of his clothes. The contact may keep him calm.

Change the baby's clothing on a flat surface, as in this way he is supported and your hands are free. If he is very troublesome, try putting him on your lap.

DRESSING THE BABY

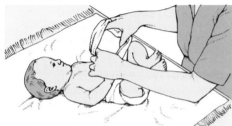

1 Place the baby on a changing mat or soft rug on a flat surface. Using an envelope-neck vest, put your fingers in the neck and stretch it as wide as possible; put it carefully over her head, avoiding her eyes.

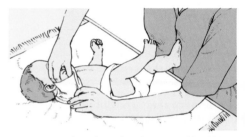

2 Put your hand up the sleeve and hold her arm gently to guide it through. Do the same with the other arm and pull down the vest as far as it will go. Use this method for any garments that go over the baby's head.

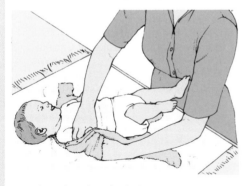

3 When dressing the baby in a stretch suit, spread it out with the front uppermost and place the baby on top. Put your hand up the sleeve, gathering up the fabric if necessary, and guide her arm through the sleeve. Do the other arm in the same way and pull the suit over her shoulders.

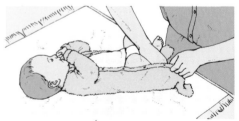

4 Gently push the baby's right leg down the leg of the suit so that her foot fits neatly into the foot of the suit. Do the same with the other leg and do up the poppers.

Undressing the baby
Put the baby on a flat surface, then follow the above steps in reverse. Take care to keep the clothes clear of the baby's eyes. Wrap her up in a warm towel immediately, so she does not get distressed.

SELECTING CHILDREN'S CLOTHING

The new baby

Mothers of new babies are often given far too much clothing, most of which their babies rapidly outgrow. The rule is to keep clothing simple: avoid fussy garments; use flame-resistant fabrics where possible.

Vests with envelope necks slip easily over babies' heads. One-piece garments are practical and warm, but do not misunderstand the term "stretch suit". This type of garment is intended to stretch only within the age range for which it is specified and will not grow with the baby.

Raglan sleeves make dressing and undressing easier. Lacy garments are best avoided as there is a danger of small fingers becoming trapped in holes. Draw-strings should also be avoided. Buttons should be securely fixed as loose ones can be swallowed or pushed into the nose or ears. If a baby is kicking vigorously, especially at night, with the result that he is cold and uncovered, a sleeping-bag outfit is very practical. Warm outdoor clothing in winter is essential, especially for the head, from which heat is lost rapidly (see page 105).

Clothes for the new baby

Toddler clothes

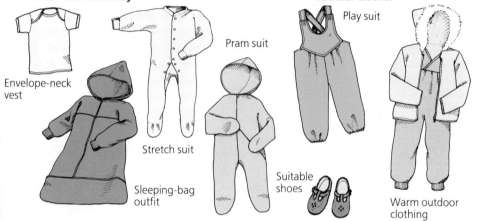

Envelope-neck vest

Stretch suit

Pram suit

Sleeping-bag outfit

Play suit

Suitable shoes

Warm outdoor clothing

The older child

It is outside the scope of this book to discuss clothing for children in detail, but some general principles apply: clothing should be roomy, with wide armholes and plenty of legroom, lightweight while suitable for the time of year. Tight bands and belts are best avoided: garments that fasten in the front make it easier for a child to learn how to dress himself. Stretch fabrics are practical and comfortable. Buying new clothes one size too big is a false economy: when they are new they do not fit properly, and by the time they fit they are wearing out.

Shoes

A young child does not need shoes until he is walking out of doors. Before this going barefoot will allow his feet to develop without damaging restriction, and give him a better sense of grip.

Shoes for everyday wear should preferably be made of leather and be at least 1.5cm longer than the child's foot. The front end should be very wide and rounded, not pointed. Lace-ups are best as they give most support, though well-made sandals are cool in warm weather. Proper fitting and checking of all shoes is essential.

EATING AND DRINKING

HELPING THE PATIENT TO TAKE AN ADEQUATE DIET AND FEED HIMSELF

Food and drink are necessary to life and health. They also give a great deal of pleasure. Everyone enjoys good food, attractively served in pleasant surroundings. Even the ill person whose appetite is not large will often respond to an attractive meal served to him at the right time.

If you are concerned with preparing and serving food to a patient, it will help you to understand the basic principles of good nutrition. You should know how the body uses food, what nutrients are needed in a balanced diet, and in what foods they are found. This knowledge will help you to prepare balanced meals according to the needs of the patient. If you also take care to present meals attractively so that they look appetizing, you have a good chance of overcoming any reluctance of the patient to eat caused by the loss of his appetite.

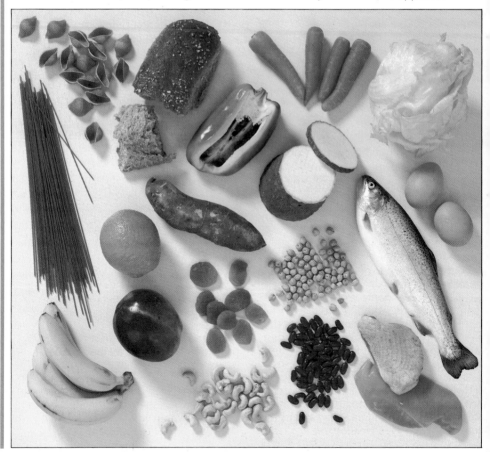

THE IMPORTANCE OF HEALTHY EATING

To eat well means to eat a variety of foods containing the different nutrients, which are the basic substances that the body needs to remain healthy. The nutrients in food are used by the body:

■ to provide energy for movement
■ to provide heat so that the body temperature remains stable between 36°C and 37°C
■ to provide for normal growth
■ to replace cells as they wear out or are destroyed by illness.

The principles of good nutrition are based on knowing a person's needs and on satisfying them with foods containing these essentials. The dietary needs of the individual differ according to age, sex and occupation. Children and young people need more protein for growth; men need more food than women; the young and active use more energy and need more food than the elderly or those who lead a quieter life; the manual worker uses more energy and more food than the typist. Climate is also a factor: in cold weather, people need more food to keep warm.

Bearing in mind these broad principles, you can work out the right quantity of food for a particular person. Dieticians calculate food requirements in a scientific manner, using the joule as their unit of measurement: 4.8 joules equals 1 calorie. For practical everyday eating, exact calculations of food requirements are unnecessary. What matters is that the diet should be varied and interesting.

Elements in a balanced diet

Ideas of what constitutes a balanced diet have altered from believing that sources of protein in the form of meat and dairy produce were the most important elements, to putting much greater emphasis on wholemeal bread, potatoes and fresh vegetables. This is due to a better understanding of the effects of fibre, sugar and

fat on our bodies and to changes in our lifestyle. We eat less than we did years ago, we are not as physically active and the balance of our food has changed: we eat less bread but the same amount of fat, for example. In general, we tend to be overweight and eat too much fat, sugar and salt, and too little fibre.

Fibre is the part of plant food which passes through the body unchanged. It adds

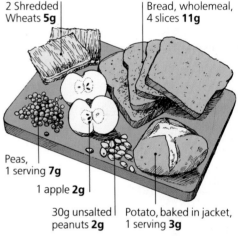

2 Shredded Wheats **5g**

Bread, wholemeal, 4 slices **11g**

Peas, 1 serving **7g**

1 apple **2g**

30g unsalted peanuts **2g**

Potato, baked in jacket, 1 serving **3g**

One 30g portion of fibre
All adults should aim to eat at least 30g of fibre a day. This illustrates how easily that amount can be made up with widely available foods.

bulk to the diet and helps to prevent or alleviate many bowel problems. Most of us eat only about half of the 30g of fibre we need each day. Eating extra fibre is satisfying and so helps to reduce the fat and sugar intake.

Fats are high in calories and are often a major factor in excessive weight gain. Some fats are necessary to the body: they are a concentrated source of energy and contain fat soluble vitamins. Saturated fats are linked to a high incidence of heart disease as they raise the blood cholesterol, which in

CATEGORIES OF NUTRIENT

Nutrient	In which food	Importance to body
Proteins 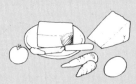	Meat, fish, poultry, eggs, milk, cheese, peas, beans, nuts, cereals, tofu.	Proteins are necessary throughout life for the replacement of worn-out cells. They also promote growth, so they are essential for pregnant women and children. During a long illness or after a serious operation the body is severely deprived of protein. The body cannot store protein, so some must be eaten daily.
Carbohydrates	Potatoes and some other root vegetables; bread, flour, cereals, rice, pasta. Sugar and all products sweetened with it (such as sweets, biscuits, cakes, puddings, ice cream and jam).	All starches and sugars are broken down into glucose by the body to provide heat and energy. They are essential in moderation, but excess is turned into fat.
Fats	Butter, margarine, cooking fat, cooking oil, lard, dripping, meat fat, cream, milk, cheese, egg yolk, olive oil, fish oils, salad cream, mayonnaise.	Fats are a concentrated source of warmth and energy. People tend to eat fatty foods more in the winter, but it is easy to take them in excess at any time: a summer meal of, for example, cheese salad with lashings of salad cream contains a large amount of fat.

Vitamins

Vitamins are essential for good health and are present in many foods in minute quantities. Lack of them leads to deficiency diseases. Anyone eating a well-balanced diet will automatically take in enough vitamins. If the patient's diet is inadequate, the doctor will prescribe a vitamin supplement to compensate, which must be given daily as prescribed.

Nutrient	In which food	Importance to body
Vitamin A	Liver and fish liver oils; milk, butter, cheese, eggs, fortified margarine; can be manufactured by the body from carotene, a substance found in carrots, tomatoes, and the outer skin of green vegetables.	Vitamin A protects the body from infection and contributes to the processes of growth. A lack of it leads to diseases of the eye. It is possible to take too much vitamin A. Workers in child health clinics are alert for symptoms of overdosage.
B vitamins 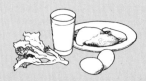	Unrefined cereals, liver, yeast, nuts, some meat, Marmite, tofu, okra, watercress.	This very complex group of vitamins has several different components. Lack of any one of them leads to diseases of the skin or nervous system, and is also thought to cause some types of mental confusion.

Nutrient	In which food	Importance to body
Vitamin C	Fresh citrus fruits, early summer fruits such as strawberries, guava, papaya, mango, potatoes and some green vegetables such as the outer leaves of cabbage.	Vitamin C aids the body's healing power. It cannot be stored in the body so must be taken daily. Without it a condition known as scurvy arises, which can prove fatal if not recognized and treated. A number of elderly people who live on a diet of tea, bread and butter may suffer to a mild degree from the disease.
Vitamin D	Eggs, fish liver oils; can be made by the body when the skin is exposed to sunlight, although this source is only reliable in certain countries.	Vitamin D is essential for the proper use of calcium and phosphorus in the body; lack of it leads to a disease of the bones known as rickets. It is possible to have too much; parents who give children cod or halibut liver oil should not exceed the stated dose. Workers in child health clinics are alert for symptoms of overdosage.
Vitamin E	Wheatgerm, milk, cereals, nuts, egg yolk; liver.	Vitamin E helps to protect the body's cells from damage and degeneration.
Mineral salts (especially iron)	Eggs, cocoa, liver and baked beans; sprouting seeds – mung, aduki, alfalfa, mustard and cress; iron tablets. Remember to keep iron tablets in a safe place: they are brightly coloured and look like sweets but are highly dangerous to young children: if too many are taken, they can be fatal.	The body needs small quantities of mineral salts to maintain its functions and in a well-balanced diet there are enough of these. Iron, however, vital for the formation of red blood cells, is often in short supply. If the body has insufficient iron, a condition known as iron-deficiency anaemia results. This is common, especially in pregnant women.
Water	Some water is taken in when liquids are drunk and when food is eaten, since many foods, especially fruits and vegetables, contain high proportions of water.	Water is vital to life. The body is 70 per cent water: nearly all body tissues contain water and many glands produce quite large quantities of watery secretions. Water is constantly being lost from the body: through the skin, the air breathed out and the elimination of urine and faeces. Many people do not drink enough fluid every day.

turn can build up inside the artery walls especially around the heart, causing blockage and eventually a heart attack or heart disease. Polyunsaturated fats are safer in this respect but the calorie value is the same.

Sugar can cause dental decay and lead to weight increase. Sugar contains calories but no other nutrient. Try to reduce intake of

sweets, cakes and chocolate, and avoid products with added sugar. Use artificial sweeteners, unsweetened fruit juices, low calorie drinks and "unfrosted" cereals.

Salt is necessary to the body in small quantities, but most of us eat about ten times more than the 1g we need daily. In some people salt leads to a rise in blood pressure and this is why anyone with high blood pressure is advised to restrict salt intake. It is wise, however, for us all to reduce our salt intake.

FATS

Saturated fats are mainly of animal origin, and include:

> meat
> milk
> sausages
> bacon
> butter
> cheese
> ghee
> hard or hydrogenated margarine
> avocado
> chocolate
> meat pie
> lard
> dripping
> shellfish.

Unsaturated fats, or **polyunsaturates** and **mono-unsaturates**, are mainly from plant seeds and include:

> vegetable oils:
>> corn oil
>> sunflower oil
>> soya bean oil
>> sesame oil
>> olive oil
> soft margarine (when labelled "high in polyunsaturates")
> nuts
> ground nut oils
> oily fish:
>> herring
>> mackerel
>> trout.

Milk is an important source of protein, calcium and vitamins, but full milk contains a lot of fat. The following are the types of milk now available, with grams of fat per pint:

Ordinary or whole milk, silver top	**11g**
Semi-skimmed, red and white top	**5g**
Skimmed, blue top	**1g**

Hidden sugars

We consume far more sugar in our food than ever before, mostly in the form of hidden sugar in processed foods. The following diagram shows the amount of sugar in teaspoonfuls contained in some common foods:

Packet soup **4tsp**

Soup, small-sized tin **1½tsp**

Baked beans, medium-sized tin **4tsp**

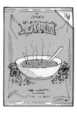 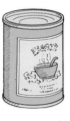 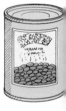

Ketchup, per bottle **27tsp**

Orange squash, per glass **4–5tsp**

Cola, per tin **7tsp**

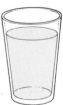 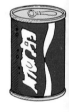

Flavoured yoghurt, per carton **4½tsp**

Honey, 1lb **100tsp**

Jelly, 2 cubes **18tsp**

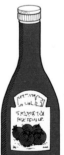 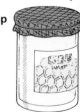

Food additives preserve or change food in some way: they may enhance the colour, texture or flavour. Their presence is listed among the ingredients of most packaged foods either by name or by a number. These numbers are helpful to those people who are allergic to certain additives and who need to identify their presence. Many manufacturers are cutting down on the additives in some products and entirely removing them from others.

Convenience foods are not all "junk foods". Frozen vegetables, for example, may contain far more vitamins than "fresh" ones that have lost their vitamin content during storage. Tinned beans, sardines, tuna fish and sweet corn are also good. Dried, frozen or unsweetened tinned fruit may be acceptable alternatives to raw, fresh fruit if that is unavailable. Frozen, pre-packaged meals, however, require careful thought. Many are high in carbohydrate and low in protein, filling but not sustaining, and not satisfactory as a balanced diet. But they are tempting for busy people who have to shop and cook in a hurry, and for elderly people who cannot be bothered to cook hot meals for themselves. Pre-packaged meals will do no harm once in a while, provided they do not become the main element in the diet and are not the only source of nutrients.

Some people eat an unbalanced diet through ignorance; others do so through lack of time, money or imagination, or through self-indulgence. Low-income groups, such as the elderly, cannot afford expensive protein foods like meat or fish, or the added cost of cooking them. They resort to the cheaper carbohydrate foods, which are easily prepared or bought ready to eat. Such foods will fill the stomach without providing adequate nourishment for the body. You may be able to advise your patient on a better diet by explaining food values and simple principles of nutrition.

For healthy eating, follow these seven general guidelines:

- reduce sugar
- reduce fat
- reduce salt
- increase fibre
- avoid overweight
- eat a varied diet
- read the labels on food packages.

Alcohol

Alcohol has become an accepted part of our normal diet. It is a pleasant social habit but can lead to problems of dependence, alcohol-related illness and sometimes overweight. Heavy drinkers suffer from deficiencies of nutrients and vitamins, and in excess alcohol acts like a poison and damages the body, especially the liver.

To keep within a safe limit a sensible intake would be:

Men   4 – 6 standard drinks,
Women   2 – 3 standard drinks,
No more than 2 – 3 times a week.

SALT

On average we consume 10g (2 teaspoon-fuls) of salt per day, although our bodies need only about 1g. We should aim to reduce the amount of salt eaten per day:

Reduce the amount of salt used in cooking and added to food;

Eat less of the following foods:

cheese
crisps
salted nuts
sausages
bacon
cornflakes
meat pies;

Look for labels saying a product has "No salt" or "No added salt".

ONE STANDARD DRINK

One standard drink is equal to:

½ pint of ordinary beer
1 single pub measure of spirits
1 small glass of sherry
1 glass of wine.

Remember that drinks poured at home tend to be more generous than those poured in bars or public houses.

NUTRITION IN ILLNESS

For a number of conditions the doctor will order a specific diet, which must, of course, be followed carefully. In many other cases, the doctor will simply indicate the type of diet to give the patient. You then have freedom of choice within the prescribed limits, according to the patient's tastes.

Fluid diets

The patient is only given fluids. An adult should have at least 3 litres (about 5 pints) a day and at least half of this should be milk. Whole, or unskimmed, milk is a unique fluid because it contains every food requirement, with the exception of vitamin C and iron. Some patients will drink milk as it is, others prefer a flavouring, such as cocoa, coffee, chocolate, malted milks or Bovril. If the patient is very thin or undernourished or if he is likely to be taking fluids only for some time, one of the protein preparations such as Complan can be added to the milk.

To complement the milk the patient may have water, fruit juice, thin soup or any other suitable drink, such as Bovril. It may be helpful to remember that since an average cup holds about 150ml of fluid, 20 cups will be needed to give the required daily intake of 3 litres (3000ml).

The doctor will advise on the amount of fluid a child should drink each day. Children may need to be encouraged and tempted to drink as much as they need to. Try diluting fruit juice, to help them drink more of it. Give them milk flavoured with milkshake mixes according to their preference, and serve their drinks in different glasses and cups, with brightly coloured straws.

Light diets

A light diet consists of easily digestible foods such as fish, white meat, eggs, milk, bread and butter. Vegetable and fruit or fruit juice are given in small quantities but fried foods should be avoided. A light diet can seem boring but a little ingenuity works wonders and attractive presentation of the food may solve the problem.

Special diets

Many special diets play an important part in the treatment of some diseases, such as diabetes. In this disease, the body is unable to store any reserves of glucose. Carbohydrates are therefore given in limited quantities, just adequate for the body's immediate needs. If the diet is not followed, the patient may become unwell and if he is then not treated he may lose consciousness and die. If you are caring for a diabetic patient, you will usually be supplied with a diet sheet but, if there is any difficulty, you should seek the advice of the doctor, community nursing sister or health visitor.

Another common special diet is the low-calorie diet, prescribed for the patient who is overweight. There is evidence that excessive or unhealthy eating habits are learned in infancy: over the years there can be a steady increase in weight. Metabolic factors may be another cause. Overweight people are much more likely to develop illnesses of various kinds, such as joint and back pain, coronary artery disease and high blood pressure. Prevention is always better than cure, and anyone who has a tendency to be overweight would be wise to restrict his total carbohydrate intake during illness or convalescence and be careful not to eat between meals: prolonged inactivity may exacerbate a tendency to gain weight. Once a diet is prescribed for someone who is seriously overweight, however, carbohydrate foods are drastically reduced. A diet sheet is prepared for the patient providing approximately 1000 calories (4000 joules) a day. Bread, potatoes and sugar are severely restricted and replaced by salads and fresh fruit. The main purpose is to re-educate the eating habits, as most people positively enjoy the carbohydrate element in their food and do not like to be restricted to items which they probably regard as unsatisfying and inadequately "filling"

FOOD HABITS

Although the diet of a healthy person must contain essential nutrients, these can be obtained in many ways and there are no essential foods. Even in a small country like Britain, food patterns vary from one part of the country to another: high tea is more popular in the north of England than in the south, for instance. It should not therefore be surprising that the food habits of people in other countries are often very different.

Food habits are established in childhood and familiar food gives a sense of security. Some men are so rigid in their habits that they will only eat food prepared by their mother or their wife. Others are reluctant to try new dishes, even though most people might accept unfamiliar food as part of the enjoyment of a holiday, for instance. For the same reasons, immigrants often find it difficult to adopt the food patterns of their new country. Religious beliefs may play as large a part in this as traditional attitudes.

A little knowledge of your patient's food habits will help you when preparing a meal, for people who have strict dietary rules may also wish their food to be prepared and stored in certain ways. Ask the patient or his relatives if this is so; if his diet is dictated by religion and you are in any doubt about it, consult his religious adviser.

Dietary rules must be respected. The Moslem is forbidden alcohol and pork, but other types of meat are acceptable provided that they have been ritually killed. Orthodox Jews have rigid food laws: meat and fowl must be killed by specialists and prepared according to Jewish law so as to be kosher. Pork, bacon, ham, rabbit and shellfish are forbidden and meat and milk products may not be eaten at the same meal, with the same crockery, or at the same table. The Hindu is not allowed to eat beef. The vegetarian never eats meat, fish, dripping, suet or fish oils, and sometimes not even gelatine or rennet – anything in fact that necessitates killing an animal; but he will eat dairy products. A vegan is a very strict vegetarian who will not even take dairy products and relies on milk, butter and cheese made from nuts or soya beans.

HELPING THE PATIENT TO EAT

A meal should be as enjoyable an occasion as possible. It is all the more pleasurable if eaten in agreeable surroundings at a well appointed table or from a thoughtfully laid tray. This applies to the sick person no less than it does to the healthy one.

THE PATIENT WHO CAN FEED HIMSELF

The patient must be comfortable. Give him the opportunity to empty his bladder and wash his hands before the meal. Make sure he is warm and well supported with pillows. When you bring the tray make sure it is clean and set with all the requirements: the patient will find it irritating to watch his meal get cold while you run for the salt you forgot to put on the tray. The food itself should be something the patient likes, and prepared to give maximum enjoyment, especially if the patient needs tempting to eat. Serve it in small portions and garnish it to make it look attractive and colourful. Give the patient time to eat each course but, as soon as he has finished the meal or eaten as much as he can, remove the tray from the bedroom so that the patient doesn't have to look at dirty dishes and unwanted food.

THE BLIND PATIENT

The blind patient is usually able to feed himself with a little thoughtful preparation, so be careful not to limit his independence. If he wishes, cut the food up into bite-sized pieces and arrange it around the plate. You can then tell him that the potatoes are at 1 o'clock, the meat at 4 o'clock and so on. If he cannot feed himself, try to avoid saying "next" or "open" when each mouthful is ready; instead tap his chin when you want him to open his mouth. This leaves you free to carry on your conversation.

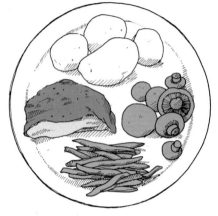

Preparing a plate for a blind person
If a blind person is told where on his plate his food is, he can select mouthfuls for himself.

THE PATIENT WITHOUT TEETH

The patient without natural teeth may find chewing difficult and need a soft diet. Prepare foods that can be mashed, and use a mincer, liquidizer or emulsifier if available. Avoid extra spices and seasoning as healed gum surfaces are very sensitive.

THE HELPLESS PATIENT

Some patients are in the unenviable position of being unable to feed themselves, so you must undertake this important task. Before the meal help the patient into a comfortable position and protect the bedclothes with a napkin. Bring the tray to the bedside just as you would to any other patient, as the sight and smell of food can still give pleasure and increase appetite. Find out the patient's preferences regarding the food's temperature and flavour.

Sit down by the patient and feed him with a fork or a spoon, allowing time for each mouthful to be properly chewed. If the patient can sit up, he can drink from a cup. If he is lying flat, give drinks through a straw or from a feeding cup (see page 68). Remember that the patient drinks from the *bottom* of a feeding cup first so make sure there are no tea leaves or coffee grounds in the drink. Turn each mealtime into a pleasure: chat to him while feeding him, but remember not to expect him to talk back to you while he is eating.

THE UNCONSCIOUS PATIENT

When a patient is unconscious, the swallowing reflex is lost. Any food or fluid put into the mouth is likely to drain down into the lungs, perhaps causing death from asphyxiation. This is why it is so important not to try to give an unconscious or even semi-conscious person a drink — it may prove fatal. Such patients are fed either by a tube through the mouth and into the stomach or by special sterile fluids into a vein. You are unlikely to have to feed an unconscious patient.

HELPING TO PREPARE MEALS

The elderly, arthritic and disabled often find preparing meals difficult. Physical handicaps may be relieved by the provision of various kitchen aids but, in some cases, regularly prepared meals can be provided.

You may also come into contact with the patient living on his own who cannot be bothered to cook for himself. He may just need encouragement and company or he may also need regularly prepared meals.

Meals on Wheels
The Meals on Wheels service provides a regular midday meal. Ideally the service runs from Monday to Friday but, in some cases, a meal is provided two or three times a week. The service is run by the WRVS or other voluntary services as agents for the Social Services Department. Clients pay a fixed contribution each time a meal is delivered; the amount varies according to the locality. Although the service's main function is to provide a meal, it also means each client is seen daily or at regular intervals by a volunteer who is interested in his welfare. As a general rule, the Meals on Wheels services do not cater for special diets.

Day centres and clubs
Day centres and luncheon clubs are usually run by the statutory authorities and by voluntary groups. Many provide a midday meal for those attending the centre for the day, while lunch clubs often cater only for the midday meal. For more about day centres see page 144.

The Marie Curie Foundation
Patients with some forms of cancer may be eligible for special help from the Marie Curie Foundation. For instance, if the patient has difficulty in swallowing, the Foundation may fund the purchase of special food and equipment such as a liquidizer. If there is anything the patient needs, talk to the community nursing sister.

AIDS TO EATING AND DRINKING

Many aids exist to help people with different types of disability, ranging from weakness in the hands to loss of the use of one arm. Most of the aids illustrated here are designed to reduce difficulties and encourage independence among patients; some, the feeding cups, are intended for use with helpless patients.

For patients with one arm
The patient with the use of only one arm may find a plate with an integral rim helpful (right, above) or a plate guard (right, below). A combined knife-spoon (right) or a knife-fork-spoon (far right) are also excellent aids.

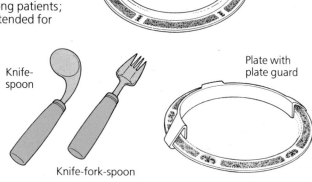

Plate with integral rim

Plate with plate guard

Knife-spoon

Knife-fork-spoon

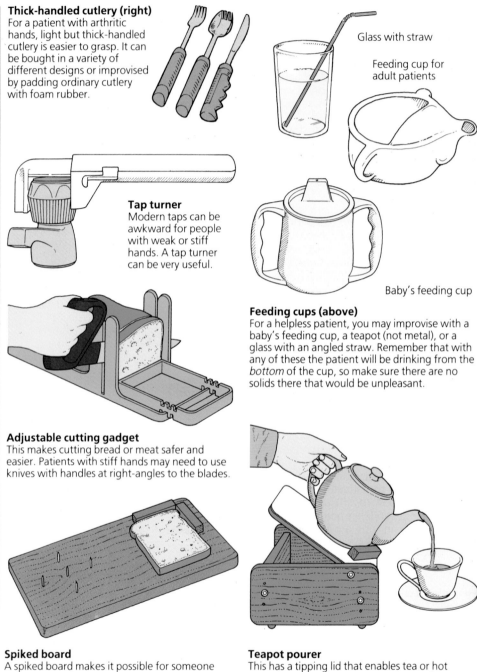

Thick-handled cutlery (right)
For a patient with arthritic hands, light but thick-handled cutlery is easier to grasp. It can be bought in a variety of different designs or improvised by padding ordinary cutlery with foam rubber.

Glass with straw

Feeding cup for adult patients

Tap turner
Modern taps can be awkward for people with weak or stiff hands. A tap turner can be very useful.

Baby's feeding cup

Feeding cups (above)
For a helpless patient, you may improvise with a baby's feeding cup, a teapot (not metal), or a glass with an angled straw. Remember that with any of these the patient will be drinking from the *bottom* of the cup, so make sure there are no solids there that would be unpleasant.

Adjustable cutting gadget
This makes cutting bread or meat safer and easier. Patients with stiff hands may need to use knives with handles at right-angles to the blades.

Spiked board
A spiked board makes it possible for someone with the use of only one hand to butter bread or peel potatoes.

Teapot pourer
This has a tipping lid that enables tea or hot water from a kettle to be poured out safely and easily. A lip prevents the pot from sliding.

MINOR DIGESTIVE PROBLEMS

Many patients confined to bed for much of the time suffer from heartburn or indigestion, while occasional vomiting is a part of several different conditions.

Heartburn and indigestion

Heartburn and indigestion are two very common problems, which cause a large amount of discomfort. Heartburn is caused by the back flow of stomach acid into the oesophagus. It is felt as a burning sensation in the centre of the chest (hence its name "heartburn"). The sufferer often feels most uncomfortable after a large meal when he is lying down or bending over to pick something up from the floor.

Indigestion is most commonly the result of unwise eating. Rich or spicy foods, excessive alcohol or smoking can all cause a temporary inflammation of the stomach lining. The patient has a sensation of fullness and discomfort in the upper abdomen, which is sometimes accompanied by belching and nausea.

The best way of preventing heartburn and indigestion is to avoid giving the patient large, rich or spicy meals, or foods he doesn't like. Alcohol should be taken in moderation and not on an empty stomach. Smoking should be restricted.

The acid in the stomach can be neutralized with a glass of milk or a mild antacid tablet. Warm milk is particularly effective at night. Sit the patient up if the discomfort is severe. Do not give a strong antacid (or any antacid over a long period) without the doctor's consent. If the patient is suffering from a great deal of flatulence, peppermint water sipped slowly is very effective. If pain persists or recurs, inform the community nursing sister or the doctor.

Vomiting

Vomiting is distressing for the patient, especially if it happens without warning.

If a patient starts to vomit, fetch a bowl immediately. Remove any false teeth if you can. Steady the bowl. If the bedclothes have soiled, cover them with a paper towel while the attack lasts. When it is over give the patient a mouthwash and wash his face and hands, before changing his bedlinen and clothing as necessary.

Observe the amount and character of the vomit. Unless it is either water or undigested food, save a specimen for the doctor. Place this in a covered jar and keep it in a cool place away from the patient. Flush the remaining vomit down the lavatory. Observe the patient's colour and pulse rate. Make a note of:
■ the time of vomiting
■ whether the vomiting is associated with eating or drinking
■ whether pain is associated with the vomiting (in some conditions pain is relieved by vomiting; in others it increases).

Leave the bowl, washed and covered with a cloth or towel, near the patient's bed in case he vomits again.

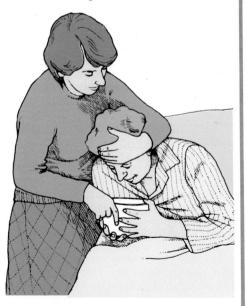

Vomiting in the patient confined to bed
Support the patient's head over a bowl while she is vomiting; afterwards freshen the air.

FEEDING THE NEW BABY

Deciding whether to breast or bottle-feed is one of the major decisions every new mother has to make and most mothers – particularly with their first baby – will want advice. This should be readily available from someone with knowledge and experience, such as the midwife or health visitor.

The wishes of the mother are as important as the needs of the baby. Whichever method is adopted, satisfactory infant feeding depends on a contented baby and a happy mother.

BREAST-FEEDING

Breast milk is quite different from cow's milk. It looks rather like water, and indeed many mothers think that their milk is "no good for the baby" because it looks so watery. This is not the case: breast milk is meant to look exactly the way it does. It also contains valuable antibodies. As long as the mother is eating well, the baby will receive all the nutrients he needs in his first months.

Breast-feeding is easier than bottle-feeding. The milk does not need to be sterilized, nor does it need to be warmed. It does not have to be specially stored, nor does it have to be prepared before use.

When to feed
Many mothers prefer the idea of fixed feeding times. During the first weeks of the baby's life, however, they will be lucky and unusual if their baby also prefers fixed feeding times! Demand feeding usually turns out to be more satisfactory for both mother and baby. Instead of keeping a crying baby waiting for his next feed, or waking a sleeping baby when it is "time" to feed him, the baby is fed when he is hungry.

In fact, babies who are on a self-demand schedule usually acquire a routine of their own. Feeding times will rarely be evenly spaced but will nevertheless be found to occur at about the same time every day.

All babies need feeding at night for at least their first six weeks of life. Some persist in wanting an extra night feed for weeks or even months. In these circumstances, patience is the only solution. The baby will not go on wanting to be fed at 2am or 3am

for ever; in the meantime it would be unfair to refuse his demand.

How much to give
There is no accurate way of telling how much milk a baby takes when he is breast-fed. For some mothers, this uncertainty is one of the strongest inducements to bottle-feed. If, however, a mother can be persuaded to continue with breast-feeding, within a very short time she will know well enough whether or not her baby is satisfied.

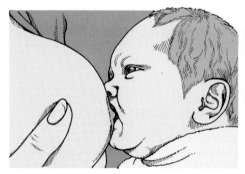

The position of the baby
The baby should feed with both the nipple and the surrounding area in his mouth for the best flow. Make sure he has room to breathe, and that his head is above the level of his stomach.

How long to take
Feeding time is not merely an opportunity to get food into the baby. Mother and baby need to get to know each other and to build up the ties that come from the physical contact of feeding.

As a general rule, about ten minutes sucking at each breast is adequate, but it is usually recommended that one breast at least is emptied at each feed. It is customary to start the feed on alternate sides. Some babies get all they want from one breast, others need only five minutes on each side. Others still are only content if they are allowed twenty minutes or more at each breast. A new mother will be given advice about how long to take over feeds from the hospital or her health visitor, and she will soon learn to know when her baby has had enough at each feed.

POSITIONS FOR FEEDING
A comfortable position, plenty of time and – especially in the first weeks – all the privacy you need are the basic requirements for giving satisfactory feeds. Hold the baby so that his head is well supported.

Alleviating mothers' anxieties
Many mothers want to breast-feed, but feel that their supply is inadequate. In the first few days after birth this is quite normal. After that nature usually achieves a perfect balance between the demands of the baby and the mother's ability to satisfy him.

There are no specific foods or fluids which will improve the mother's supply of milk. Neither are there any special medicines which are known to help. A mother who really feels worried that her baby is not thriving because she has not got enough milk should take expert advice.

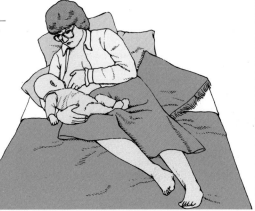

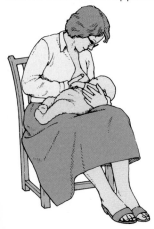

Sitting up
The ideal chair for nursing is low, upright and armless. It provides good support for the back, as long as the baby is correctly positioned – perhaps with the help of a pillow.

Lying propped up
If you choose to feed your baby lying down, make sure that most of your weight is taken by pillows. You will soon feel tired if you spend the feed leaning on your elbow.

BOTTLE-FEEDING

If a mother is really unhappy at the prospect of breast-feeding her child, or if in exceptional circumstances she proves unable to do so, bottle-feeding is a perfectly adequate and acceptable alternative.

Choice of bottle and teat
Feeding bottles can be made either of glass or of plastic. For convenience, measurements of volume are marked on the outside.

The shape of the sucking end of the teat resembles the human nipple as nearly as possible. The teat should have a hole large enough to allow milk to drip out unaided when the bottle is held upside down, at a rate of several drops a second. If an existing hole is too small, it can be enlarged by piercing the teat with a red-hot needle (placing the eye of the needle in a cork before heating it will prevent burnt fingers). Sterilize the teat before use.

Choice of foods
There are many varieties of milk on the market that are suitable for feeding babies – and a few that are not. Giving unmodified milks to babies under six months old is dangerous. Formula milk should be used until the baby is at least six months old.

Formula milk is the usual substitute for breast milk, and is cow's milk adapted specially for babies to make it resemble human milk. In dried, powder form formula milk can be bought from many food shops, child health centres or chemists, and there is no significant difference between any of the standard dried milks. Liquid formula is also available, although less readily.

Sterilizing feeding equipment
In preparing any type of food for a baby, contamination with germs must be avoided. All utensils must be sterilized and you should wash your hands before you start.

Immediately after use all bottles and teats should be rinsed inside and out with cold water, washed in warm water with washing-up liquid, then rinsed again. The teat should be rubbed inside with salt to remove any milk that may have got trapped and rinsed thoroughly once more. Bottles and teats should then be immersed in a container filled with sterilizing solution. It is important that no air bubbles are trapped inside the bottles or teats. If you have not bought a purpose-made container, you may need to cover the teats with glass to stop them floating to the top. Leave the bottles and teats in the solution for at least two hours before draining. Rinse with cool boiled water.

It is also possible to sterilize feeding equipment by placing it in a saucepan of warm water and boiling for three minutes.

STERILIZING THE BOTTLES

1 Immerse all the bottles and teats in warm soapy water. Scrub the insides with a bottle brush kept specially for this purpose. Rub salt inside the teats to remove all traces of milk. Rinse bottles and teats thoroughly in warm water.

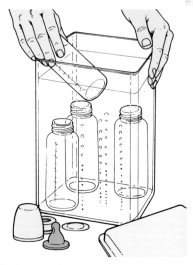

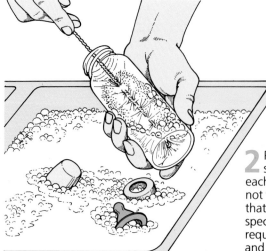

2 Put the bottles, teats, measuring jug and spoon into the sterilizing tank, holding each item under until it is full so that it will not float. Trap the teats under glass. Ensure that everything is fully submerged for the specified time. Take each item out as required, drain the excess back into the tank and rinse the item with cool boiled water.

Bottles for the baby

The number of bottles you have will depend on how you organize your sterilizing. Even if breast-feeding, one or two bottles will be needed for giving water or juice. Milk should flow from the teats at the rate of several drops a second, and should feel warm, not hot, when splashed on to the inside of your wrist.

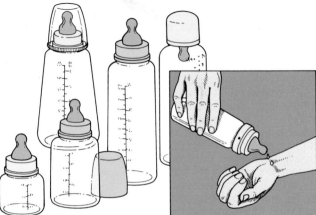

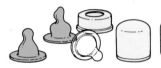

Preparing bottle-feeds

Before you start, clear a working surface or spread out a clean towel. Collect everything you need, making sure that all bottles and teats are sterile. Wash your hands. Follow exactly the instructions on the packet or tin of formula milk, but if in any doubt, check with the midwife or health visitor. If you are using a liquid formula, you should wash and sterilize the top by pouring boiling water over it before opening.

Many mothers find it convenient to make up a day's supply of bottles and store them in the refrigerator. If the baby doesn't want it all that day, throw the left-over milk away and make up more the next day.

MAKING UP A POWDER FORMULA

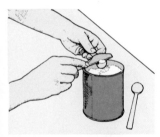

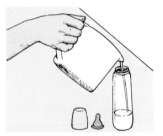

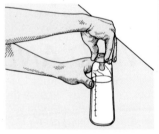

1 Boil the kettle. Use some of the cooled boiled water to rinse the equipment from the sterilizing unit, then fill the measuring jug with the correct amount of water. Check it at eye level. Scoop out the milk powder, levelling each scoop off with the back of the knife, and add to the measuring jug.

2 Stir the solution thoroughly with a sterilized spoon to make sure the powder dissolves in the water completely. Fill the bottles with the formula, according to how much is calculated for each feed. Check the measure at eye level. Never add any extra formula to the measuring jug or the bottles.

3 Put the teats, upside down, into the bottles and screw on the lids; or put covers over the teats, depending on the type. Put all the bottles in the refrigerator immediately, and store them for no longer than one day. Stop the bottles falling over by standing them on a small tray or in a plastic box.

How to give a bottle-feed

Either place the bottle with its teat and cover in a jug of hot water, or leave it standing until it reaches room temperature. Wash your hands and sit in a comfortable chair. Support the baby just as if you were breast-feeding (see page 71). Before giving the feed shake a little milk on to the inside of the wrist – don't use the palm of your hand to test it, because the skin there is used to hot temperatures and will not be sufficiently sensitive. The milk should be comfortably warm, not hot. Hold the bottle downwards to keep the teat full of milk, not air. If the baby does not want the whole bottle, throw the left-over milk away: do not keep it for a later feed.

The aim of bottle-feeding is to make it as like breast-feeding as possible. The same relationship needs to be established, so the mother should feed the baby herself whenever possible. The baby needs to feel the same closeness and security that it would when breast-feeding.

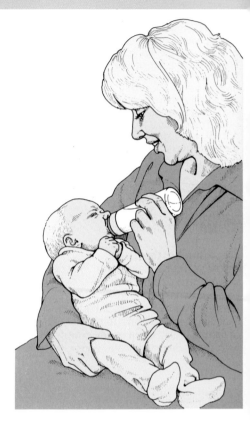

Bottle-feeding the baby

Physical contact is just as important to the bottle-fed baby as to the breast-fed one: hold him and smile at him while giving a feed, as if breast-feeding. Make sure the teat is full of milk, not air.

WIND AND COLIC

Whether breast- or bottle-fed, most babies get wind. This is because their sucking is not completely efficient and some air is gulped in with the milk. Usually mothers find it best to pause halfway through a feed, take the baby from the breast or remove the bottle and put it down, and place him against her shoulder or upright on her lap while gently patting his back.

Some babies cry regularly between 6pm and 10pm feeds every evening. This can be

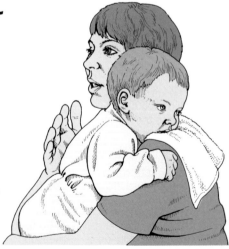

Bringing up wind

Some babies bring up a little milk along with air when they burp. This is quite normal, but a sensible mother usually protects her clothing.

very disturbing for both parents, but it usually stops spontaneously when the baby is about 13 weeks old: thus it has been given the name "three-month colic". What causes it is not clear, nor why it happens in the early evening. Time usually improves

matters without other help. Babies who cry persistently and frequently, however, apparently from some kind of pain in the abdomen, have rarely just got wind: in most instances the baby has real colic and expert advice is needed.

WEANING

The addition of solids to a baby's diet is called weaning and is usually begun at about four months and completed by nine months. Only very small amounts are given at first to introduce new flavours, prevent digestive upsets, and get the baby used to the idea of solid food.

The kind of food given depends on whether or not the baby can chew. Most babies begin to chew at about six months, even if they have not yet got any teeth. Before the baby can chew he must be given foods which can be swallowed as they are. These could be pre-cooked baby cereal, fruit or vegetable purées, gravy (especially from fresh meat), grated cheese, egg yolk (not egg white as this can produce allergies in very young babies), mashed banana and even very finely minced meat. There are many proprietary baby foods, cereals and desserts on the market and these are quick and easy to give, but where possible fresh foods are preferable.

Each food must be introduced in a small amount. A teaspoonful twice a day is adequate at first and if the baby refuses that particular food it should not be offered again for several days. The stools should be

observed for signs of digestive upsets.

Once the baby can chew, the variety of foods can be increased. By his second year he will be able to have almost anything that is being served at a family meal.

Special dietary problems
Children may in relatively rare cases require special diets. A few babies are allergic to the protein in cow's milk and have to be given foods prepared from goat's milk. Some older children are found to have sensitivity to gluten, a protein found in most cereals and grains. These children fail to thrive at any time: after weaning they lose weight and pass large fatty stools. Once all gluten has been eliminated from their diet improvement is speedy. However, wheat, rye, barley and oats will probably have to be excluded from the diet for life.

Parents of children who are apparently not thriving or who are showing signs of sensitivity to certain foods should act under medical supervision only. Tests will have to be done and a detailed diet sheet provided, and a mother should be discouraged from experimenting with her child's diet without proper medical supervision.

FEEDING THE SICK CHILD

What a child eats when he is ill should be regulated by his appetite. Fluids are important, especially if he is vomiting or has diarrhoea. Clear fluids are best, such as water, plain or flavoured. Milk may make vomiting worse and is not advisable for babies with diarrhoea.

In short illnesses of a week or less there is

no need to encourage the appetite with specially prepared tit-bits. A small helping of a child's normal diet will be acceptable. On the other hand, in a prolonged illness the child should be encouraged to take foods essential for growth, health, and repair to diseased tissue: that is, a diet rich in proteins and vitamins (see pages 60–1).

MEDICINES

HELPING THE PATIENT TO TAKE AND CARE FOR HIS MEDICINES

The ancients were studying simple plants for their healing properties long before anything precise was known about the nature of drugs. The plants were used to prevent disease, cure illness or relieve symptoms, but nothing was known about their mode of action.

It is only in recent years that the study of drugs has developed into a highly exact science. The simple plants have been analysed and their active principles have been found. Research workers have found ways of producing many of them synthetically, so reducing their cost and increasing their purity. The number of drugs has increased, and the action of many is exceedingly powerful – so much so that there is now a range of conditions caused by the drugs themselves. Many drugs have side-effects: examples are the drowsiness that results from taking a sea-sickness pill or the weight gain that sometimes comes from taking the contraceptive pill.

Because of their potency and the possibility of side-effects that might be harmful, it is vital that drugs are given only to the person for whom the doctor prescribed them. No patient should ever be allowed to use up a drug originally prescribed for somebody else.

If you are looking after a patient in the home, you may be called upon to give him medicines. Medicines may contain one drug or more. As long as you exercise due care, give only what the doctor ordered, and follow four basic rules, errors should not occur. These are the four basic rules:

1 Check the medicine is the right one.
2 Give the exact amount ordered.
3 Give it to the patient for whom it was prescribed.
4 Give it at the time ordered by the doctor. If you want to remember these easily and quickly, think of them as giving:

■ the right amount
■ of the right medicine
■ to the right patient
■ at the right time.

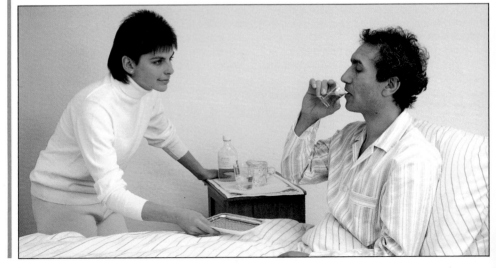

GIVING MEDICINES

Medicines can be given by mouth – whether in the form of tablets, capsules, liquids or powders – by injection, by inhalation, or via the rectum; those designed to treat a specific condition locally may be applied to the skin, or instilled into the eyes, nose or ears. Ensure a prescribed course of treatment is followed to the end, particularly penicillin or antibiotics. All medicines should be stored safely (see pages 80–1).

MEDICINES BY MOUTH

The most usual way of giving drugs is by mouth. Medicines given by mouth come in several forms. They may be liquids, tablets, capsules, pills or powders. You will proceed slightly differently according to the type of drug you are giving. Always follow the doctor's or pharmacist's instructions on whether a particular medicine should be given before or after food.

Before you start to give any type of drug by mouth, prepare a small tray. On it should be a glass of water, the drugs you need, and a clean medicine glass or 5ml spoon.

Giving tablets, capsules or pills
You must first check the bottle or box by reading the label. Shake out the correct number of tablets into a spoon and read the label again. Give the tablet to the patient in the spoon, accompanied by a glass of water. Make sure he swallows the tablet. Some tablets are very large and may be difficult to swallow, or the patient may have difficulty: if so, tell him to place the tablet towards the back of his tongue. Sugar-coated tablets, capsules and pills must be swallowed whole. They are coated either against an unpleasant taste or are meant to dissolve slowly in the stomach. Uncoated tablets may be divided into smaller pieces with a knife or crushed between two spoons, provided that the doctor approves.

Giving liquids
First check the bottle by reading the label. Check the dose and expiry date. Place your index finger over the top, and shake the bottle well. Remove the top and put it on the tray, inner side upwards. Hold the bottle label uppermost, so that any drips while pouring will not obliterate the instructions. Hold the glass at eye level and measure the dose ordered. Replace the screw cap or cork and read the label again as a double-check. Give the dose to the patient on a tray, and make sure he drinks it. Afterwards wipe any drips off the bottle and wash the medicine glass or spoon.

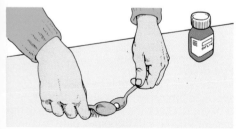

Crushing uncoated tablets
If the patient finds swallowing uncoated tablets difficult, crush them up between metal spoons so that he can either swallow the powder with water, or take it in a spoonful of jam or honey.

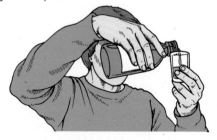

Measuring the dose
Hold the bottle with its label uppermost, so that any drips will not obliterate the instructions. Hold the medicine glass *at eye level* and accurately measure the dose ordered.

Giving powders
You can either mix the powder with jam or honey or stir it into a small quantity of milk or water and give it to the patient at once.

It is important to remember that if the patient is being given a special diet, any milk, jam or honey should be considered as part of that diet.

MEDICINES BY OTHER ROUTES

Drugs by rectum
Drugs given this way are given as suppositories or retention enemas. They are inserted into the rectum and the patient is asked to try to retain them. The drug is absorbed slowly and the effect lasts for several hours. See pages 87–8 for more about how suppositories and enemas are given.

Drugs by inhalation
Drugs given this way are added to steam and take the form of an inhalation (see page 128). Alternatively the patient may be provided with an aerosol or inhaler containing the relevant drug, which he can use for himself when he needs to. Such drugs are intended to relieve breathing in conditions such as asthma or bronchitis (see page 129).

Drugs by injection
Injections will normally be given by the doctor or professional nurse, but you should know that there are various types of injection. Subcutaneous injections are injected just under the skin; intramuscular are injected rather deeper into muscle; intravenous are injected into a vein.

Diabetic patients needing to have regular injections will be taught how to inject themselves by a professional nurse or doctor. You

Injections for children
With a child, tell him that he will feel a prick in his arm, then try not to let him look at the needle while the doctor gives the injection.

may need to check that they have had their injection at the correct time. Parents of diabetic children may be taught how to give the necessary injections until the child is confident enough to give his own.

DROPS

Eye, ear or nasal drops are supplied in small bottles fitted with droppers, in little plastic containers or even as a single application. Some are dangerous if taken by mouth. Eye drops are supplied sterile, and should be used within a limited period after opening: always check if this is the case. In addition there may be an expiry date, which must be observed irrespective of the date on which the drops are opened.

Eye drops
Most eye drops may only be used for a specified time after the seal has been broken, so check the instructions. Check the patient's name and the expiry date.

Check also if the drops are to go into one or both eyes. This is important: many eye drops are prescribed for a specific eye and may cause serious damage or even blindness if put into the other eye by mistake.

Ask the patient to sit down and wash your hands. Stand behind him and ask him to look up. Hold the dropper horizontally, with your hand resting on his face. Apply slight pressure to the lower eyelid to bring it away from the eyeball and insert the drop gently into this space, near the outside corner of the eye. Let the eye close and ask the patient to blink. This spreads the drop over the whole surface of the eye.

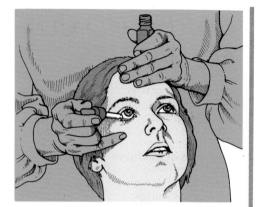

Administering eye drops
Hold the dropper horizontally, taking care not to touch the patient's eyes. Ease the lower eyelid away from the eyeball and insert the drop.

Ear drops
Check the patient's name and the expiry date. Warm the drops, where allowed, by standing the container in a bowl of warm water. Protect the patient's clothing with a paper towel and wash your hands. Ask him either to lie down, or sit with his head tilted, so that the affected ear is uppermost. Rest the tip of the dropper just above the ear and allow the drops to trickle down into it. Ask the patient to keep his head in the same position for a few minutes.

Nasal drops
Check the patient's name and the expiry date. Wash your hands. Lay the patient down on his back so that his head is hanging over the edge of the bed. Alternatively, sit him down and tilt his head back as far as possible. Insert the tip of the dropper just inside the nostril and allow a drop to go in. Repeat on the other side. Ask the patient to sniff. If he is lying across the bed, ask him to stay there for a few minutes for maximum effect.

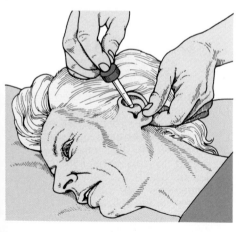

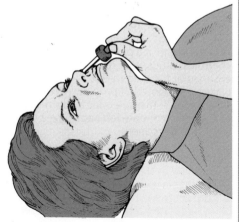

Administering ear drops
Make sure that the patient's head is tilted with the affected ear uppermost. With the tip of the dropper resting just above the ear, let the drops ooze gently in. The patient should not move his head for a few minutes after the drops have been inserted, to prevent them running out.

Administering nose drops
Ideally the patient should receive nasal drops lying across a bed on his back with his head hanging down over the edge. This position is uncomfortable, however, and some may find it unpleasant. The patient may therefore prefer to sit down and tilt his head well back.

CARE AND CUSTODY OF MEDICINES

Most accidents connected with drugs occur in the home because of carelessness. In hospitals and institutions stringent rules exist for the care and custody of drugs.

Categories of medicine
Drugs fall into several categories: general sale medicines that can be bought in any shop or supermarket; pharmacy medicines which can only be sold under the supervision of a pharmacist; and drugs obtainable on prescription only.

Among the substances obtainable on prescription from a doctor only are the controlled drugs. These are substances which make the taker dependent on them, and they include strong pain-killers such as opium, morphine and heroin; sleeping tablets such as temazepam (Normison); and stimulants such as amphetamines. All are taken "for kicks" by drug addicts.

Stringent legislation controls the ordering, storage and use of these drugs in hospital. If you are undertaking hospital duties, you must make yourself familiar with hospital rulings.

In the home, if a patient of yours is taking controlled drugs, your responsibility is to ensure that the drugs are stored in a safe place and disposed of properly when the time comes. If they are tablets, check and record how many are left each time a dose is given to the patient.

Storing medicines
If you abide by the following rules, drugs will be safe in your care.
■ Keep drugs for internal use in a safe place, separate from substances intended for external application.
■ Never transfer medicines from their original bottles to other containers.
■ Never mix different sorts of pills and tablets in the same container.
■ Keep medicines in a cool place: the doctor will tell you if any drug needs to be stored in a refrigerator.
■ Do not use any medicine if you cannot read its label clearly.

Deterioration of medicines
Drugs deteriorate and it is necessary to be able to recognize substances unfit for use.
■ Do not give drugs or drops that have passed their expiry date.
■ Do not give any substance, liquid or solid, that has changed colour.
■ Do not give an originally clear liquid that has become cloudy or has developed a sediment that was not there before.
■ Do not give if you cannot read the label.
■ Do not give a drug if anything raises a doubt in your mind about giving it.

Disposing of medicines
When a drug is no longer required it should be flushed down the lavatory. If a patient has died, dispose of any drugs he was taking without delay.

DISPOSAL OF SYRINGES

If a disposable syringe was used to give an injection, place both the syringe and the needle in a strong cardboard box or appropriate hospital container and keep safely until full, when it will be collected by the community nursing sister or health authority van. Local arrangements may vary slightly. This will prevent the refuse collector from being injured and drug addicts from getting hold of a used syringe.

GIVING MEDICINES TO CHILDREN

If medicines have been prescribed for a child by a doctor, the child needs those medicines. He should take them, even if he dislikes them or if he seems better.

Most children take their medicine quite readily. Liquid medicines are often prescribed for small children, in which case you should have a glass of the child's favourite drink ready to wash the taste of the medicine away after he has taken it. If the child really dislikes the taste of his medicine, you can disguise it by mixing the medicine with a spoonful of jam or honey. Do not pretend to the child that you are only giving him jam: he will notice the drug and will not trust you again. Tell him that it is his medicine but that it will not taste unpleasant if he takes it this way.

Keeping medicines safe
It is important not to confuse medicines with sweets for another reason: the child may get the idea that all pills are nice to eat, especially if he has been used to taking suger-coated coloured pills. Many iron pills, for instance, are perfectly safe in the recommended dose, but they look like Smarties and children may swallow them in handfuls: they can cause death.

Every medicine should be regarded as potentially dangerous to children. Some are more dangerous than others, but no tablets are completely safe if too many are swallowed. For this reason medicines should not be kept within reach of small fingers. They should be locked in a safe cupboard with the key kept somewhere different, not left in the door. Medicines to be kept in the cupboard should include *all* substances containing drugs: these include skin creams and menthol for inhalation, not just liquids and pills.

Because of the dangers, medicines today are dispensed with safety in mind. Bottles have "childproof" tops and tablets are packed in plastic and foil strips. These are excellent deterrents for children, but can cause problems for the elderly or those with weak or arthritic hands. If medicines are always kept in a locked cupboard, safety tops are not strictly speaking necessary, but there is never any harm in taking extra precautions.

In any normal household there are many ordinary products which are also potentially dangerous. Experience has shown that the following are particularly hazardous: ammonia; antifreeze liquid; brake fluid; caustic soda; oven cleaner; paintbrush restorer; paint stripper. It is better to be safe than sorry. Keep these substances and any others that are similarly not intended for internal use under lock and key and in a high cupboard that is well out of the reach of children: they should *not* be kept in the cupboard under the kitchen sink, however convenient that may be for you.

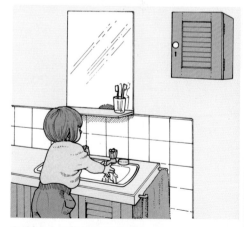

Storing medicines out of reach
A medicine cabinet should be well out of a child's reach and above her eye level, so that she is less likely to be interested in it. If it is also kept locked with no key visible, you can be fairly sure that the child is safe.

ELIMINATION
HELPING THE PATIENT TO DEAL WITH HIS EXCRETIONS

Helping the patient with elimination is one of the most testing aspects of your nursing care. A difficult and embarrassing service for the patient to accept, he must never sense that it is difficult or embarrassing for you to give. Your priority is to maintain the patient's dignity at all times, even if he is unconscious, and to provide privacy.

The normal elimination from the body is from the bladder, the bowel and the skin. Women also lose menstrual fluid from the vagina. The patient may vomit (see page 69) or have a cough and produce sputum (see page 130). These excretions are often saved, as they may provide valuable information about the patient's condition.

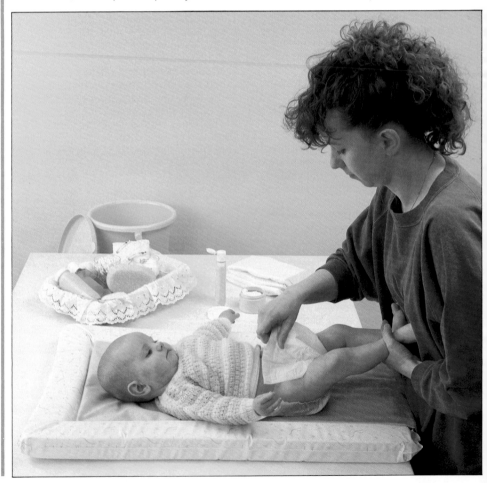

BASIC CARE

To attend to the patient's needs satisfactorily, you must know how much he is able to do for himself and when he is likely to need help. He may be able to walk to the lavatory, perhaps with just a steadying hand from you; but he may not be able to go as far as the lavatory, in which case he may either be allowed out of bed in the bedroom to use a commode or have to use a bedpan or urinal in bed.

The patient must be given the opportunity to follow his usual habits. Most people tend to pass urine soon after they get up in the morning and many have been in the habit from childhood of passing urine before a meal and before going to sleep at night.

USING A COMMODE

Make sure the bedroom door is closed before helping the patient out of bed. Put his slippers on for him and place a dressing gown or shawl around his shoulders. If necessary, help the patient to move his pyjamas or her nightdress out of the way, then seat the patient carefully. Cover his legs with a blanket: this muffles the sound of urine and reduces embarrassment, both from the sound and from exposure. See that there is a toilet roll within the patient's reach and leave him in peace – unless he is weak or unsteady, in which case remain nearby. Afterwards encourage him to wash his hands; if it is not possible for him to walk as far as the nearest basin, have ready a bowl of water, soap and a towel for his immediate use. Help him back into bed. Cover the pan and empty it down the lavatory; rinse in cold water and replace. Wash your hands. Eliminate smells with an air freshener, and return the room to normal as quickly as you can.

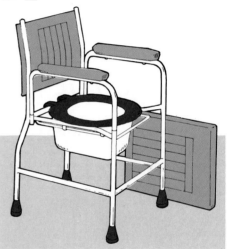

A commode
This type of commode is in common use in hospitals. Often used in homes is the type that looks like an ordinary chair (see page 17).

GIVING A BEDPAN

Make sure the bedpan is warm and dry before taking it to the bedside covered with a paper towel or piece of kitchen roll. Also take a toilet roll. Make sure the bedroom door is closed to ensure privacy. Help the patient to lift up her nightdress or slide down his pyjama trousers. Use one hand to help him raise himself while you slip the pan under him with the other. (If he is allowed to sit upright against pillows, the whole procedure is easier and more natural.) After he has finished, let him use the toilet paper, unless he is too ill to manage when you will need to attend to this for him. Take the pan away from him and cover it immediately. Rearrange the nightclothes and bedlinen and make the patient comfortable. This is often a good opportunity for changing his position in the bed, and so helping to prevent pressure sores (see page 29).

Let the patient wash his hands while you take the covered pan to the lavatory and rinse it with cold water. Wash your own hands. Return to the bedroom and use an air freshener to eliminate unpleasant smells.

Male patients will only require a bedpan for a bowel action. They should be given a urinal at the same time, as well as when they only need to pass urine.

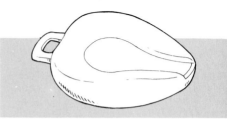

A polypropylene bedpan
This type is now in common use in homes and hospitals, and is cheap to buy.

GIVING A URINAL

Cover the urinal with a paper towel or a piece of kitchen roll, take it to the bedside and hand it to the patient. If he is very ill or helpless, place it in position. After use, cover it, empty it and rinse it in cold water.

Many men have difficulty in passing urine lying down; whenever possible they should be allowed to stand by the bedside. If a urinal is not available, a wide-mouthed jar is a good substitute.

AIDS IN THE LAVATORY

Various aids exist to help the elderly and disabled to use the lavatory by themselves.

They may be of great help to frail, arthritic, paralysed or elderly people.

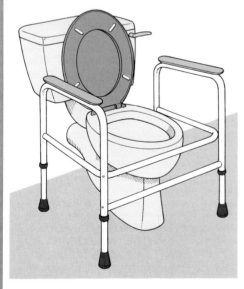

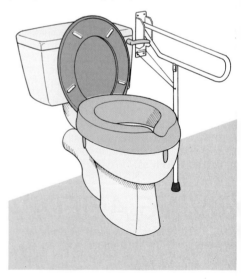

Lavatory frame
A frame around the lavatory may help patients with weak limbs, or those who need help to lever themselves up or down.

Wall-mounted handle and raised seat
A simple wall-mounted handle will help some patients to get up from the lavatory. A raised plastic toilet seat may also help patients who have difficulty in sitting down low.

URINE

The two kidneys filter the blood and produce urine from the waste products extracted. The urine passes down two tubes, the ureters, into the bladder. As the bladder fills it stretches, and nerve impulses are communicated to the brain signalling that the bladder is full and must be emptied. The urine is then passed through the urethra, which is a small tube that connects the bladder to the surface of the body. Normally a person can control this act.

Saving a specimen
To save a specimen of urine, collect it in a clean, dry bedpan or urinal. Pour some into a clean, dry bottle or jar with a tight-fitting cork or a top that you can screw tightly. Label the bottle with the patient's full name and address, the date and time of collection and the nature of the specimen.

You may be asked to save specimens of urine over a 24-hour period. On the appointed day when the patient first empties his bladder, discard the urine. After that, each time the patient passes urine in the course of the day, put it into a polythene or glass jar or bottle with a suitable stopper. The last specimen to go into the jar is the urine first passed by the patient the following day. Again, label the jar with the patient's name and address, the date of collection and the nature of the specimen.

Measuring output
It is sometimes necessary to know exactly how much urine the patient is passing. A jug that measures fluid in millilitres or fluid ounces should be kept in the lavatory for this purpose. The patient can pass urine into the jug or you can pour urine from a bedpan or urinal into the jug. Note the quantity of urine and write this down, together with a record of the time the urine was passed. Every day at the same time, total and record the quantity. As the urinary output is influenced by the amount the patient drinks, fluid intake is also often measured and recorded.

The urinary system

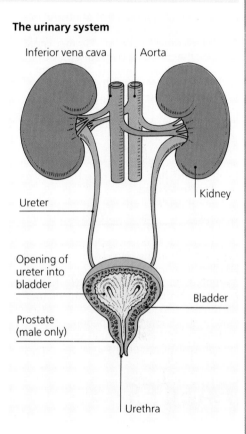

- Inferior vena cava
- Aorta
- Kidney
- Ureter
- Opening of ureter into bladder
- Bladder
- Prostate (male only)
- Urethra

Urine testing
In illness there may be obvious changes in the urine and these should be carefully noticed and recorded.

Colour: Urine is normally yellow, but it may become dark if it is concentrated, or much paler if the patient is drinking a great deal. Certain drugs may also alter the colour.

Appearance: Normally urine is clear, but the presence of certain abnormalities may make it cloudy.

Smell: Some infections or drugs (for instance, antibiotics) may cause urine to have a distinct odour. If it is left in contact with the air for any length of time it smells of ammonia.

Quantity: Normally a person passes about 1500ml of urine a day, although this quantity is affected by the amount of fluid drunk. In some illnesses, the patient may pass very small quantities of urine and in extreme cases none at all. This is a grave sign which must be reported immediately. On the other hand, in some diseases the output of urine is increased; the patient feels thirsty and drinks extra fluid.

Frequency: In certain conditions urine is passed at abnormally frequent intervals and may disturb the patient's rest at night. This should be reported.

Pain: The patient may feel some pain on passing urine or discomfort before starting to pass urine. If this is the case the doctor should be informed.

If any abnormality in the urine is observed or suspected, report this to the doctor and save a specimen for him.

It is possible to discover the presence of abnormalities in the urine by chemical tests, which have now been made very simple. In normal circumstances it is unlikely that you would be asked to test urine, but you may see it being tested by the doctor or nurse, or in some conditions by the patient.

The common abnormalities found in urine are protein, blood, sugar, acetone, bile and pus. If these substances come into contact with certain chemicals they react in a typical and obvious way, and their presence can be confirmed. The chemicals are incorporated in small sticks of card and the testing is done by dipping the stick in the urine and waiting to see if the stick changes colour. If the urine is acid, for example, the blue card will turn pink; if it is alkaline the pink card will turn blue. If neither changes colour the urine is neutral.

Explicit instructions and colour charts are supplied with every set of sticks. As long as the instructions are carefully followed the patient's urine can be tested simply, quickly and accurately.

Testing a baby's urine

The doctor might ask you to test a baby's urine if the napkin is dry when he calls. In these circumstances he will have the necessary equipment, and will give you a stick to press against a freshly wet (not merely damp) napkin. Remove it immediately, wait for about half a minute, then compare the colour of the stick with the colours on a chart and tell the doctor when he returns.

FAECES

The process of food digestion begins in the stomach and is completed in the duodenum and small intestine. Nutrients are absorbed through the intestinal wall into the bloodstream. Water and undigested remains pass into the large intestine, where most of the water is reabsorbed. The remaining wastes, known as faeces, are expelled through the anal sphincter.

Normal stools are brown in colour and semi-solid in consistency. Any deviation from the norm should be noted and a specimen saved for the doctor to see.

Saving a specimen

If possible the patient should not pass urine at the same time as faeces when a specimen

The digestive system

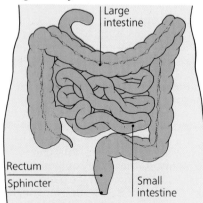

Large intestine

Rectum

Sphincter

Small intestine

is to be collected. With men this is simple as urine is normally passed into a urinal. It is generally necessary to ask women to pass urine first, before emptying and washing the bedpan and bringing it back again.

Wear disposable plastic gloves if available. Using a spatula, scoop some faeces into a waxed carton or screw-top jar. Label the container with the patient's full name and address, the date and time of collection, and the nature of the specimen. Wrap the gloves and spatula in newspaper before burning or putting in the dustbin. Empty and clean the bedpan.

DIARRHOEA

When a patient passes stools at frequent intervals he is said to have diarrhoea. The material passed becomes liquid and in severe cases may consist of coloured watery fluid. If diarrhoea persists, the patient suffers from loss of fluid, known as dehydration, and may become very ill. Diarrhoea must always be reported to the doctor without delay. Diarrhoea is particularly serious in a baby or young child as dehydration occurs very rapidly and the baby can die in a matter of hours.

CONSTIPATION

The opposite of diarrhoea, constipation occurs when the bowel does not empty itself at its usual rhythm so the stools become dry and hard. Individual habits vary: some people normally pass two stools a day, while others may pass only one every 48 hours. Constipation occurs when the normal pattern is disturbed.

Constipation in the healthy person
In an otherwise healthy person constipation may be the result of not drinking enough fluid, not eating enough fibre or not allowing enough time for a bowel action. Fibre, which stimulates the bowel, is found in fresh fruit and vegetables, in cereals (especially unprocessed bran or porridge) and in wholemeal bread (see page 59).

Correction of diet and habits will often relieve constipation. Medicines known as aperients are extensively advertised and widely used to speed up normal bowel movement and so cause an evacuation.

They have no effect on the cause of constipation, however, and therefore the condition persists.

Constipation in the patient
When people are ill they often become constipated. This may be the result of restricted diet, of increased fluid loss from sweating, or simply of unaccustomed inactivity. The patient may also be reluctant to drink in an attempt to avoid bedpans.

You should assess the patient's condition and respond accordingly. Encourage him to drink more, unless for any reason fluids are restricted. Add water, fruit juice and fibre to the diet. Give him a bedpan or help him to the commode at a time when he would normally have a bowel movement. Above all, be sensitive to his feelings and his dignity: ensure his privacy and, if possible, leave him undisturbed.

If nothing else works the doctor may order a suppository or an enema.

SUPPOSITORIES AND ENEMAS

Giving a suppository
A suppository is cone-shaped and solid, and is a way of administering a drug into the rectum. Because it is made of a substance that melts at body temperature, the suppository melts when placed in the rectum, but will also melt in the hand if held for too long.

Start by washing your hands and tell the patient what is to happen. See that he has passed urine before you begin. Help him to lie on his left side and draw up his knees. Ask him to relax by breathing deeply in and out through the mouth. Remove the foil from the suppository and put on a rubber glove or fingerstall. Dip the suppository in warm water before inserting it gently into the rectum and pushing it up as far as possible. If two have been ordered, insert the second in the same way. Remove the glove or fingerstall and place it in a paper bag before burning it or putting it in the dustbin. Wash your hands.

Encourage the patient to retain the suppository for as long as possible before using the commode or bedpan. After a bowel action has taken place, report on the stool, noting its colour, size and consistency.

Certain drugs are given in suppositories

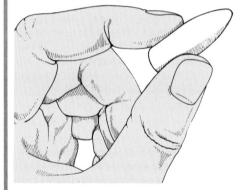

A suppository, approximately actual size.

as a treatment, and they are absorbed through the rectal wall into the bloodstream. These suppositories must be retained in the rectum so no bedpan is given afterwards. The patient should be encouraged to pass urine beforehand.

Giving an enema

An enema is an injection of fluid into the rectum, usually given with the intention of stimulating a bowel movement. A disposable enema has the fluid contained in a small plastic bag and a rectal nozzle attached ready for use. Before use it should be warmed.

Start by washing your hands and tell the patient what is to happen. Help him to lie on his left side with his knees drawn up. See that he is adequately covered and place a paper towel on a piece of plastic under his buttocks to protect the bed. Ask him to relax by breathing in and out through his mouth. Break off the tip of the nozzle and smear the nozzle with petroleum jelly. Insert it gently into the rectum for 8–10cm, taking care not to damage the rectal wall. Gently squeeze the bag, so injecting fluid into the rectum. Withdraw the nozzle into a paper tissue or kitchen paper.

Encourage the patient to retain the enema for as long as possible before using the commode or bedpan. After a bowel action has taken place, report on the stool, noting its colour, size and consistency. Wrap the enema apparatus in newspaper before burning it or putting it in the dustbin. Wash your hands.

MENSTRUAL FLUID

Most female patients of childbearing age continue to menstruate when they are ill. You will need to see that a supply of sanitary pads, along with a belt or protective pants, is available, or tampons if preferred. If the patient is not allowed out of bed, she may find it difficult or impossible to insert a tampon, so pads may have to be used.

Every time a bedpan or commode is used, provide a paper bag for the soiled sanitary

pad. If the sheets get stained, the patient may be extremely embarrassed. Change them with the minimum of fuss and soak in cold water or biological detergent.

The patient may suffer discomfort or pain (dysmenorrhoea), particularly if she is normally active. A well-protected hot water bottle (see page 107) and a mild pain-killer (analgesic), if allowed, will usually be adequate treatment.

INCONTINENCE

Difficulty in the control of the bladder or bowel can occur at any age if there has been damage to the area or to the brain. The involuntary escape of urine or the emptying of the bowel is a very distressing and humiliating experience, and it is not surprising that people suffering from incontinence often isolate themselves.

URINARY INCONTINENCE

The bladder is a muscular bag, the outlet of which is guarded by two circular bands of muscle. A small baby has no control over this muscle and its bladder empties immediately and involuntarily. As we grow and the nerve pathways develop, we learn to control the muscle. From then on we are conscious when the bladder is full and have the control to wait for a convenient place before passing urine. It is when something disturbs that control, such as infection, injury or degeneration, that we become once more unable to control the muscle: this is known as being incontinent.

Incontinence in children
The child who has gained control over his bladder may become incontinent because of some interruption in the normal pattern of development. There may be a physical cause or an emotional one. Parents usually find it very distressing and clinics exist to help the family to overcome the problem.
   Another worry is the child who is exceptionally late in gaining control over his bladder. Many children develop slowly and parents often forget how difficult it is for a child to accept enforced delay, even after he has gained control of his bladder. Staying dry at night is often seemingly impossible to achieve, and may take some time. If consistent incontinence is going on up to and beyond the age of eight years, parents would be wise to seek medical advice.

Stress incontinence
Many women suffer from stress incontinence, especially after childbirth. This means that whenever sneezing, coughing or laughing raises the intra-abdominal pressure, urine escapes involuntarily, causing embarrassment and discomfort.
   The condition is due to the stretching of the ligaments and muscles that support the womb (uterus). The womb drops and in so doing presses on the bladder. This is known as a prolapse, which may have to be cured by an operation.

Incontinence in older men
The older man may sometimes find it difficult to pass urine even though his bladder is full (a condition known as retention of urine). This is because the prostate gland, which encircles the top of the urethra (see page 85), has become enlarged and is making it difficult for urine to get past. The bladder becomes overfull and eventually urine dribbles out (retention with overflow). This type of incontinence can also be treated by an operation.

Incontinence in the physically handicapped
Anyone who has damage to the spinal cord and who is a paraplegic has lost control of his bladder. Emptying of the bladder is therefore involuntary and intermittent. Some of these patients eventually re-learn control, but some have to rely on incontinence aids permanently (see pages 91–2).

Incontinence in the elderly
By far the largest group of sufferers from incontinence are the elderly. They may lose control of the bladder or their decreased mobility may simply make it impossible for them to reach the lavatory in time.
The inability to wait: Urgency may be the result of infection, which the doctor may

treat with antibiotics. The problem may also be one of mobility. Old people need to get to the lavatory quickly when their bladders are full. If their movements are too slow, accidents occur. Some old people have arthritic hands and find adjusting their clothing difficult. Consider this when buying new clothes (see pages 53–5). Regular visits to the lavatory (especially after meals), walking aids, and, if possible, a room near the lavatory will all help.

Patients with speech difficulties may be unable to ask for a bedpan.

True incontinence: This means that all bladder control is lost. The brain no longer controls the function and the bladder acts as it does in the baby: it empties suddenly, frequently and involuntarily. The loss of control may be only temporary: after a minor stroke, for instance, control is eventually regained; but after severe brain damage, loss of control is permanent.

FAECAL INCONTINENCE

Inability to control the bowel is a rarer problem than losing control of the bladder. It may be caused by a bowel infection or, occasionally, by a severe psychological disturbance (most common in childhood). Another cause is severe constipation, when an accumulation of faeces partly blocks the intestinal passage. If it is so severe that the faeces begin to decompose and become fluid, frequent and involuntary bowel movements occur as the more liquid faeces seep past the obstruction and leak out. The condition can be successfully treated with diet and fluids.

HELPING THE INCONTINENT PATIENT

A great deal can be done to help the incontinent patient who, already humiliated and distressed, must not also be made to feel a nuisance. The bladder tends to respond to a routine, so a regular visit to the lavatory every two or three hours may help. An alarm clock or kitchen "pinger" can be used as a reminder. Patients should be encouraged to drink, for cutting down on fluids makes the condition worse, not better. However, it is sensible to control fluid intake late in the day.

It is important to avoid constipation: include fresh fruit, vegetables and fibre in the patient's diet every day.

When urine is passed involuntarily, attend to the patient promptly. Wash and dry the skin thoroughly but gently, and apply a waterproof cream. If the patient is up and about, special pants with disposable liners can be used, but these may not be a satisfactory full-time solution as plastic causes sweating, which can lead to

soreness. During the night, absorbent drawsheets and pads may be advisable. A urinal or commode can be left near the bed for the patient's use.

Supplementary benefits are available for extra expenses associated with incontinence, such as laundry, heating, bedding replacement, floor coverings or special clothing. Many areas run a laundry service for the incontinent patient, washing and drying (but not ironing) bedlinen, nightclothes and underclothes. Collection and delivery are arranged on a regular basis.

Where incontinence cannot be treated, personal protection is essential. To feel dry and confident of being odour-free is a morale-booster. Clothing is described on page 55, while machine washable shoes or plastic shoes that can be scrubbed help to prevent odour. Advice and many aids can be obtained through the family practitioner, community nursing sister or health visitor (see pages 91–2). Unfortunately, many patients and relatives are too embarrassed to seek advice. They tend to isolate themselves as the laundry piles grow higher.

As a volunteer you can do much to make people aware of the help available. You may also be in a position to help and encourage relatives who feel incontinence is a problem to be tackled only by professionals, and are therefore reluctant to admit any responsibility themselves for supporting the patient.

AIDS FOR THE INCONTINENT

Any aid recommended should be chosen with the individual needs of the patient in mind. These will vary depending on whether the patient is incontinent only at night or in the daytime too, and on whether he is up and dressed or in bed for most of the day. The age and condition – physical and mental – of the patient should also be taken into account.

Urinals for men are especially valuable at night or when the patient cannot be moved. Female urinals are small and light. They hold 600ml and can be slipped between a patient's legs without her hips needing to be raised off the bed. A Feminal consists of a plastic holder and a polythene bag. Specially moulded to the female shape, it can be used sitting or standing and is small enough to be carried in a handbag. If the bag cannot be emptied immediately after use and a new bag attached, it can be tied and kept for a while.

There are many types of incontinence pants suitable for men and women. Fitted pants are made of a soft material with a waterproof pouch on the outside. The urine passes straight through the pants to be absorbed by a pad placed in the pouch, so leaving the skin dry. The pants are worn with the pouch opening in front: to insert the pad double it over your hand and slide it into the pouch. This is made easier if the patient's knees are apart and the pants pulled down a little. Place the pad well in front for male patients and nearer the back for women. Change the pads as required

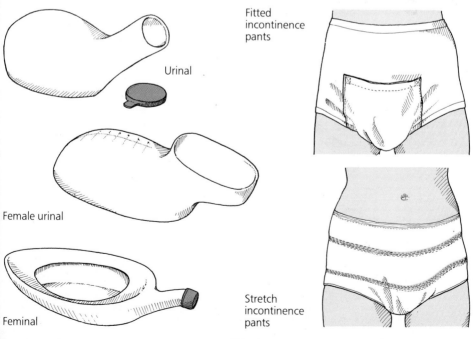

Urinal

Female urinal

Feminal

Fitted
incontinence
pants

Stretch
incontinence
pants

and the pants daily. The pants may be hand or machine washed but should not be bleached. They are not suitable for being worn at night.

Stretch pants are light, open-stretch pants designed to fit any patient, whatever their size. Across the pants are two woven-in blue bands which hold a plastic-backed pad firmly in place. These pants can be used at night and can also be either hand or machine washed but not bleached.

Underpads for use on the patient's bed are made of layers of absorbent material backed by waterproof material. There are various kinds. Pads are useful at night.

A Kylie bed sheet combines a drawsheet with an underpad. The central part is a soft absorbent yellow quilted material while the edges are thinner sheeting for tucking in. The centre allows urine to spread across it. The sheet may be left under the patient for 12 hours. It never feels really wet, just damp when saturated. It looks and feels pleasant and can be frequently laundered. A spin dryer is needed, though, as their absorbency makes these sheets heavy and extremely slow to dry. Unfortunately, they are expensive and you would need at least two.

The use of pants and pads as incontinence aids should not mean that regular visits to the lavatory are abandoned.

Dispose of soiled pads or pant liners into a plastic bag, never put them on an unprotected floor. The plastic bags for the disposal of incontinent or surgical waste may be provided through the local health authority. The community nursing sister will advise you how to get hold of them.

To give the patient more independence a catheter may be inserted into the bladder and left in position. This is known as long-term catheterization. The urine drains into a bag strapped to the leg or supported by a waist belt. The bag is emptied periodically. The problem is that catheters encourage infection. Catheters must be changed regularly by a doctor or nurse and the area around them must be kept clean. Follow the advice of the community nursing sister: she may suggest washing carefully around the catheter with soap and water, using a flannel kept for this purpose only; or the patient may be given a daily bath.

Some male patients are fitted with rubber sheaths (condoms) attached to tubing which drains into a bag attached to the leg.

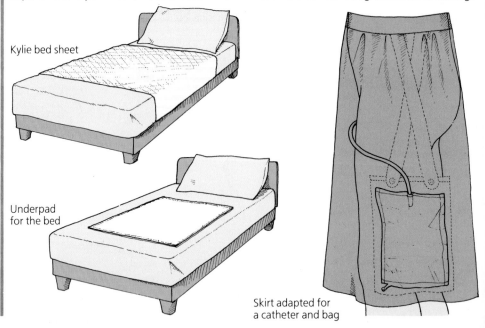

Kylie bed sheet

Underpad for the bed

Skirt adapted for a catheter and bag

THE PATIENT WITH A STOMA

In the treatment of certain diseases of the digestive tract, it may become necessary to remove part of the tract. Whenever possible the two cut ends of the tract are sewn together to maintain a passageway for food and waste materials. When this is not possible, an artificial opening (or stoma) is made in the abdominal wall through which waste material can pass into a bag.

The position of a colostomy

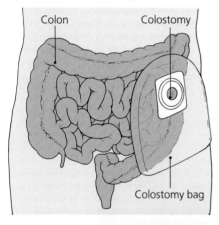

Colon   Colostomy

Colostomy bag

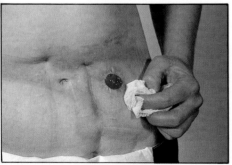

Colostomy

A colostomy is when the contents of the colon are made to bypass the rectum and the colon is brought on to the surface of the abdomen. The faeces then pass through an opening in the abdominal wall. They are fairly firm and their consistency can be controlled with diet and medicines. The patient may wear a bag and belt underneath his clothing, but once the stools are formed and regular, he may manage with just a dry dressing over the opening, exchanging this for a bag only when a bowel movement is expected. A well-regulated colostomy acts once a day: the patient can deal with it as if it were a normal rectal opening and then forget about it.

Ileostomy

The ileostomy is when part of the small intestine, the ileum, is brought on to the surface of the abdomen. This is much higher up the gut than a colostomy and the faeces passed are much more fluid. The patient requires a bag permanently in position; it must be leak-proof, unobtrusive under clothing and easy to deal with.

The stoma
When the intestine is brought on to the surface of the abdomen to create a stoma, a small section of gut is left protruding. The colostomy bag fits over this, and may be worn permanently. Some patients wear a special belt that supports the bag, others use a type of bag that attaches to the skin around the stoma with an adhesive flange.

HELPING TO CARE FOR A STOMA

Anyone seeing a stoma for the first time may feel revolted by it. This includes the family, the volunteer and the patient. Everyone feels distaste for the abnormal, and the idea of faeces being discharged on to the abdominal wall is abnormal.

The patient is distressed because he lacks bowel control; he is anxious in case he gives offence through odour or by soiling his clothes and he is embarrassed in case his appliance shows through his clothing. Relatives and friends may not be quite sure how to treat the patient: should you ignore the condition or try to offer sympathy? A simple acceptance of the situation often helps the patient most. The volunteer should be sensitive to the patient's feelings and in no way show any distaste. Gentle and confident handling will make the patient feel that this is a routine procedure and no more unusual than giving a bedpan.

Before leaving hospital, a suitable appliance is selected. Advice will be given about skin care, control of the diet, and the disposal of bags. Once controlled, the stoma should present no special problem as long as it is attended to once a day.

Ensure that the patient can deal with his stoma in privacy if he cannot go to the bathroom. He will need a bowl of warm water, soap and a towel to wash and dry the surrounding area; he should also have a paper bag in which to dispose of the full bag, and a fresh one to take its place.

When the patient has finished, remove the tray and dispose of the faeces by cutting across the top of the bag and emptying its contents into the lavatory. A pair of scissors should be kept separate for this purpose; they should be washed and dried after use. The bag can be wrapped in newspaper, burned or placed in the dustbin. In many areas special chemically treated boxes are supplied for the used bags; when the box is full, it can be sealed and placed in the dustbin. Give the patient a fresh bowl to wash his hands when he has finished.

Patients become very skilled at adjusting their own diets and protecting their skin from damage. If there are any problems consult the family doctor or community nursing sister. There are also specialist societies who can give help and support (see *Useful Addresses*).

CHANGING THE COLOSTOMY BAG

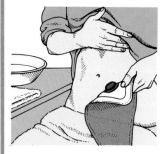 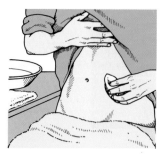 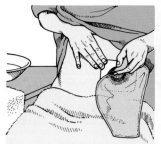

1 The patient places everything she will need on a tray near her. She removes the full colostomy bag and disposes of it into the paper bag.

2 With warm water and soap she washes the stoma and the skin of the surrounding area. Washing is important to prevent soreness.

3 After she has dried the stoma and surrounding area thoroughly with a towel, she has a new colostomy bag ready to put in position.

CHANGING THE NEW BABY

Babies pass urine frequently and should never be left in a wet napkin. Some babies pass urine at regular times but most do not. Every time you change the napkin you should wash the buttocks with soap and water, or with baby lotion, if preferred. You should then dry them well and apply a protecting and soothing baby cream before putting on a clean napkin.

Stools
Before a baby is born its gut is full of a dark green sticky material called meconium. This is passed within a few hours of birth and continues for about three days, after which time it becomes light brown in colour and is known as changing stool. On about the fourth or fifth day the stool takes on a curdy bright yellow appearance. Breast-fed babies continue to pass soft stools, while bottle-fed babies pass stools which are more solid and formed, smell more like ordinary stools and are usually passed less frequently than those of the breast-fed baby. Once weaning commences, the stools change again, becoming still darker in colour and firmer.

Napkin rash
In certain circumstances the baby's buttocks may become red and sore. It is important to change napkins frequently, to wash and dry the baby's buttocks carefully, and to rinse out napkins adequately every time. Diarrhoea may also be a cause of sore buttocks. The application of a soothing cream, such as zinc and castor oil cream, helps to protect

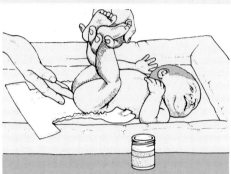

Changing a baby's napkin
Hold her ankles together with one hand while you lift her buttocks up to slide under the clean napkin and apply zinc and castor oil cream.

the skin with a waterproof layer while soothing the sore area. If none of these precautions seems to make any difference, you should seek the advice of the family practitioner or health visitor.

Types of napkin
The main decision is whether to use washable napkins or disposable ones. There are advantages and disadvantages associated with both.

The basic washable napkin is usually a terry towelling square, quick-drying but highly absorbent when folded to the baby's shape. Muslin squares can be used for very new babies and as napkin liners later on. Disposable "one way" napkin liners are now more commonly used, however: they

Disposable napkins

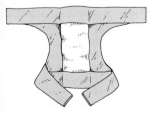

Tie-on with separate pad

Popper pant with separate pad

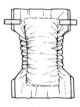

All-in-one with elasticated legs

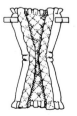

All-in-one with shaped legs

let urine through in one direction only and so protect the baby's skin.

Disposable napkins are absorbent pads with plastic backs. They are less absorbent than washable napkins, but they are certainly convenient if washing or drying facilities are limited. No napkin liners or plastic pants are necessary. Brands differ in their shapes, so find the most suitable.

Plastic pants

Plastic pants are usually used with towelling napkins. Although plastic pants are effective in keeping moisture off clothing, they tend to encourage redness and soreness. Plastic pants become hard and unusable in time, but you can prolong their life by washing them in warm water with a little washing-up liquid. Dry them away from direct heat.

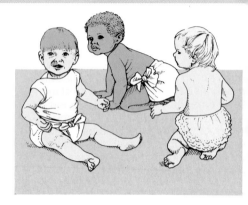

Types of plastic pants
Plastic pants come in many different designs. Those that tie at the sides are best, as they allow air to circulate.

METHODS OF PUTTING ON NAPKINS

There are many different ways of putting on napkins, depending on the sex and size of the baby. Remember never to leave safety pins open while you are changing a napkin. For added safety always secure the pins horizontally rather than vertically.

The kite method

This method is suitable for small to medium-sized babies. Lay the napkin out flat in front of you. Fold in the right and left hand corners until they meet. Fold down the top corner to make a triangle, or kite shape. Fold up the lower point a short way. Lay the baby on the napkin. Bring the lower edge through his legs and up to his waist and fasten at the corners with two safety pins.

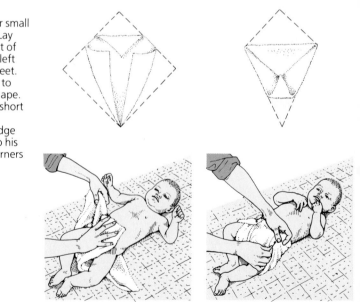

The triangle method
This method is suitable for babies of all sizes. Fold the napkin in half so that it forms a triangle. Fold down the long edge by a few centimetres, taking account of the baby's size: if the baby is small, the fold should be slightly deeper. Lay the baby on the napkin with its apex between his legs. Fold each corner around the leg and tuck under the buttocks. Pull the apex up between the baby's legs and fasten with one safety pin.

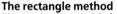

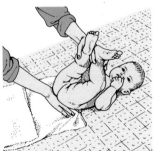

The rectangle method
This method is suitable for large or older babies. Fold the napkin in half to make a rectangle, then turn it so that one short edge is nearest you. Fold up the bottom third for a boy, or fold down the top third for a girl. Lay the baby on the napkin and bring the lower part up between his legs. Fasten the napkin at the sides using two safety pins.

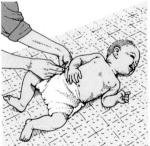

STERILIZING NAPKINS

Wet napkins must be properly washed and rinsed, so that ammonia from the urine or detergent from the wash does not come into prolonged contact with the baby's skin. Soiled napkins must be sterilized to avoid any danger of infection.

It is best to buy a special napkin sterilizing solution and two plastic buckets with lids: buy buckets of different colours or shapes or mark them so that you can tell them apart. Start by filling them both with napkin sterilizing solution. Drop wet napkins into one and soiled napkins into the other (first scraping off the worst of the soiled material into the lavatory). Do this every time you change a napkin in the course of the day. The·solution needs changing every 24 hours and to be effectively sterilized napkins need at least six hours in the solution. This means that, assuming you start in the morning, any napkins you change during the night are best stored in a plastic bag and saved for the morning's new solution.

Every morning when you change the solution, rinse out the napkins in the "wet" napkin bucket. They do not need to be washed with detergent, but they must be rinsed thoroughly. The soiled napkins must be washed in very hot water with detergent before being thoroughly rinsed. Napkins stored during the night can go straight into the fresh solution.

This method of sterilizing napkins avoids constant washing and rinsing through the day, while also saving unnecessary washing.

Napkins should be dried outdoors if possible or in a tumble dryer. If they are put to dry on radiators or hot pipes, they will become unpleasantly stiff and abrasive when put next to the baby's skin.

Napkin sterilizing solution is very strong and contains bleach. This means that coloured garments must be washed separately, even if soiled. You should also avoid any prolonged contact with the solution. Most important is never to touch the baby's delicate skin before rinsing the solution off your hands; if you find it irritates your own skin, wear rubber gloves when handling the napkins.

CONTROL OF BOWEL AND BLADDER

Managing bowel and bladder control is a skill a child learns gradually. It cannot be acquired until the nervous pathways are properly developed. Control rarely begins before the age of fifteen to eighteen months, and sometimes very much later. Some time during the second year of life a child recognizes the connection between the sensation of passing urine and faeces and the result. Control can then be learned.

Bowel control
A child's awareness of a full rectum and full bladder probably occurs at about the same time, but it is easier to "hold on" to a full rectum and bowel control is therefore likely to be achieved first. When the child makes his special movements or sounds, suggest sitting on the potty. Never force the child but let him develop at his own speed. Keep everything low key, but praise him when the desired result is achieved.

Bladder control
This is more difficult to learn and takes longer. If the child is dry after an afternoon nap, suggest sitting on the potty for a short while. Congratulate success. As soon as he is dry for reasonable lengths of time start leaving off napkins and use plastic-backed, terry towelling trainer pants, which are easy to take down in a hurry. A sudden clenching of the buttocks or standing rigid with crossed legs are usual signs of urgent need of the potty. There will be frequent puddles and accidents in the beginning. Treat these with sympathy and mop up with the minimum of fuss or the potty will be associated with tension and failure. The child may need napkins at night for a year or so and many children are occasionally wet at night until they are five. If this continues, it is advisable to consult the doctor or health visitor. When a child is ill he will often regress and temporarily lose control.

REST AND SLEEP
HELPING THE PATIENT TO RELAX AND MAINTAIN GOOD SLEEPING HABITS

Everyone is familiar with the tiredness and listlessness that commonly follow a late night. Other symptoms are headache, little interest in food and, above all, little energy to face the new day. In these circumstances, your body is suffering from the lack of sleep imposed on it.

The healthy person who sleeps well wakes up feeling physically energetic and mentally refreshed. The sick person needs more rest than the healthy one to restore energy. This is because in sickness, the body must repair the damage caused by infection, injury or disease. For this it needs plenty of rest, so that it can build up the reserves of energy necessary to fight infection and illness.

As part of your nursing care, therefore, you must make sure that the patient is getting enough sleep, so that both body and mind are relaxed. At the same time, recognize the value of rest for its own sake. Rest is restorative: a patient who finds sleeping difficult will benefit from being encouraged to relax and rest even if he does not go to sleep. The chances are, however, that a relaxed and drowsy patient will eventually fall asleep.

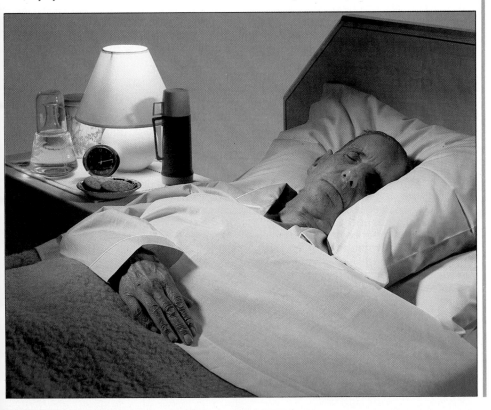

PATTERNS OF SLEEP

To help a patient rest and sleep you need to know something about his normal sleeping pattern. If he is waking up every morning in the early hours, his need for help will obviously depend on whether he usually sleeps through the night or not — early waking may be quite normal for him. You need to find out if he usually goes to bed early or late and if he is used to a nap in the afternoon. Perhaps he sleeps during the day because he works at night; perhaps he is used to a hot drink last thing at night.

It is when a person's normal pattern is disturbed that he has the most difficulty in sleeping, so learn to be sensitive to it: if you bring him a cup of tea at the very moment when he usually takes half an hour's nap, his normal pattern will be disturbed and the patient may find it harder, not easier, to get to sleep that night.

CAUSES OF WAKEFULNESS

There are many types of disturbance that can prevent a tired patient from relaxing into sleep. Some of these are practical and may prevent sleep on one isolated occasion: this type of disturbance should be relatively easy for you and the patient to identify and resolve between you. Other problems may prevent the patient from getting enough sleep night after night, without there being any obvious or simple solution. In these cases, identification of the cause is still the first step, even if this does not necessarily mean that a permanent answer to the problem is any easier to find immediately.

ENVIRONMENT

Consider the patient's environment. Is he in his own bedroom? A change of surroundings can be very disturbing, and it is not only the patient in hospital who suffers but the patient at home who is being nursed in a different room for convenience. If unfamiliarity of surroundings is keeping the patient awake, all you can do is try and leave the rest of his routine as unchanged as possible.

The patient may not be happy with the temperature of his room at night, especially if he himself is feverish. Is the room well ventilated without draughts, and are the bedclothes warm enough for the time of year without being too heavy? One blanket more or less may make a surprising difference to the patient's comfort.

Is the room free from smells? The sense of smell is heightened in illness, and the patient may be nauseated by cooking smells, stale flower water too near the bed or bedpans not removed immediately after use. The patient may even be disturbed by the smell of his own body. Discharges from a wound or stale sweat (particularly if the patient has a limb in plaster) can be extremely distressing. You can do a lot to eliminate most disturbing smells. Try not to let cooking smells linger in the kitchen or passageways. Remember to use an air freshener in the bedroom after the patient has had a bowel action. Wash his skin often, using a deodorant where appropriate, and leave a pleasant-smelling aerosol within the patient's reach so that he can use it whenever he wishes to do so.

The amount of light may disturb the patient's sleep. If his condition warrants a night nurse or night sitter, there must be a light so that she can see the patient but it should be carefully shaded to avoid disturbing him. Conversely, the child used to a small nightlight may be afraid of the darkness if he is left without one.

DISCOMFORT

People normally differentiate between night and day by wearing different clothes. It may help an ill person to feel more normal if he can also change into clean pyjamas or a fresh nightdress to sleep. Wrinkled sheets, crumbs in the bed and untucked bedclothes all contribute to restlessness. Because of this, always see that the sheets are pulled taut and smooth when you are settling the patient to sleep and that he is comfortably settled on pillows. This is especially important if the patient is totally confined to bed. The lack of any change of scene and the consequent feelings of frustration and boredom serve to intensify even the slightest discomfort. Check also that the bedclothes are not too heavy, although some patients are used to weight and miss it if it is removed – if blankets are replaced by a continental quilt, for instance.

Make sure that a patient with breathing difficulties is comfortably supported with pillows. If something is irritating his skin or there is undue pressure on any part of it,

this needs special attention (see page 29). A swollen limb may be more comfortable raised on a pillow, while painful joints are often eased if the bedclothes are supported by a bed-cradle.

A full bladder is a common cause of sleeplessness, especially if the patient is reluctant to call anyone during the night and cannot get out of bed. Always offer a bedpan or urinal when settling the patient for the night and allow plenty of time for him to use it. If he is fairly mobile, he may like to have a bedpan, urinal or commode beside him during the night.

Indigestion may be relieved with peppermint water or a simple indigestion tablet, while nausea can often be relieved with soda water. Coughing may be helped by a change of position, together with extra pillows and a spoonful of honey and lemon. If the particular discomfort that disturbs the patient *can* be alleviated by a simple remedy, the reassurance will help to relax him and prepare him for sleep.

HUNGER AND THIRST

The sick patient is often reluctant to eat and yet he may well feel both hungry and thirsty during the night. Although a large fluid intake last thing at night is probably unwise, a milky drink taken last thing before settling to sleep is often the answer. Stimulants such as tea and coffee, however, are best avoided unless the patient usually drinks these late at night.

If the patient is feverish or the weather

very hot, a jug of lemon squash or lemon barley water is refreshing. Many older people are used to a tot of alcohol at night: there is no harm in this unless expressly forbidden by the doctor.

If the patient wakes in the early hours of the morning feeling hungry or thirsty, a few biscuits in a tin or a hot drink in a thermos left on his bedside table may soothe him to sleep again.

NOISE

Noise disturbs sleep. Unfortunately, it is often those caring for the sick who make the most noise. For this reason, wear quiet shoes and clothing that does not rustle. Try to eliminate noises in cisterns and radiators if you can. Close doors quietly and make sure that they cannot swing open and

shut in a sudden draught.

Absolute quiet can also be disturbing, especially during the day, so do not eradicate all the sounds of normal living. Simply turn down the volume on the television or radio, and ask the children to play a little more quietly than usual.

FEARS AND ANXIETIES

Fear undoubtedly keeps people awake. The sick person always has fears, and it is pointless to pretend that they do not exist. In the hours of darkness they may loom especially large and seem most threatening. The patient may have many different worries: How long shall I get pay? Can we manage on sickness benefit? Shall I be fit to do my old job when I am better? Shall I get my old job back? Shall I be disfigured? Shall I still be attractive to my boyfriend or husband? Am I becoming a burden as I get older? Who will look after me when I cannot cope any longer? Shall I be able to bear the pain? Am I going to die?

All these are very real anxieties, some without solution. Yet there is truth in the old adage that a burden shared is a burden halved. Try to get the patient to *talk* to you: give him your full attention and listen properly. Most of the time you are probably so busy that you do not *really* listen. On the other hand, be careful not to pry. At night when the patient is in low spirits, he may find it possible to talk to a sympathetic listener, but the next day he may wish he had not confided in you and may not want to be reminded of your conversation the night before, or may need to be reassured that it was confidential.

PAIN

Perhaps the greatest enemy of sleep is pain. Pain can be increased by any or all of the factors discussed above, while attention to these factors will minimize and perhaps even remove the pain.

Inform the doctor of any persistent pain from which the patient is suffering. He will want to know what the pain is like, when it usually occurs and whether anything in particular seems to cause it.

Pain-killing drugs and sleeping tablets may be prescribed by the doctor to help the patient rest, but these should only be given in accordance with his instructions.

SLEEP IN THE VERY YOUNG

The new baby
A newborn baby has not yet established a sleeping pattern. He will sleep when he needs to sleep for as long as his body tells him to do so. Most babies sleep for between 16 and 20 hours a day in the first few weeks of life, but some may sleep for less time from the very beginning. He will sleep progressively less as he grows: by the end of a year he will probably sleep through the night with a nap in the morning and afternoon. During the second and third years he will take a brief nap; and by the age of five he sleeps on average about 12 hours a day.

The newborn baby tends to wake when he is hungry or uncomfortable. He does not distinguish night from day and wakes at random through the 24 hours. It takes several weeks before the baby starts to be awake during the day more than at night. He will adjust sooner if he is encouraged to distinguish between night and day from early on. Night-time feeds should be quiet and brief. He should be put down to sleep in different places: at night for instance, he may sleep in his cot, while during the day he may be in his pram in a room with a window open and with older brothers and sisters playing round him. Their noise will not keep him awake if he needs to sleep.

In fine weather the baby can sleep outside, in a sheltered spot where the sun will not shine directly on to the pram. Protect the pram with a cat net and make sure the brake is on.

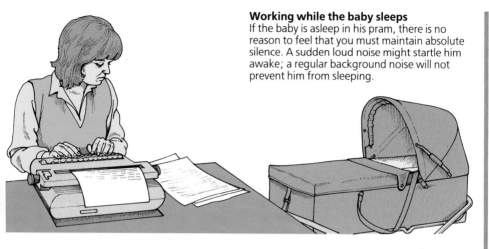

Working while the baby sleeps
If the baby is asleep in his pram, there is no reason to feel that you must maintain absolute silence. A sudden loud noise might startle him awake; a regular background noise will not prevent him from sleeping.

The sick child
When a child is feeling really ill he will lie still in bed. He will doze or sleep as much as his body dictates until he starts to feel better. All you need to do is to keep him comfortable in pleasant surroundings and give him love and attention when he is awake.

At the next stage of illness, in early convalescence, you may need to take more active steps to make sure that the ill child is getting enough rest and sleep. The child is feeling better and will therefore be more active and restless. He will be easily bored and inclined to be mischievous. He will move about as much as he can and easily become overtired, while at the same time finding it harder to rest.

It is important that at this stage you provide lots of entertainment to keep the child's mind occupied and his body rested: jigsaws, stories and as much attention as possible. If the child is busy but physically relaxed, he will sleep better at night. Even a relaxed child, however, may be kept awake by fear and anxieties, which may or may not be related to his illness.

Night fears are common in childhood anyway but they may be accentuated by illness. The sick child probably needs more comforting than usual and may have many apparently irrational fears – of the bogey man coming to take him away or of some other fantasy person in the room. Do not dismiss his fears too easily. Instead put your head down to his level and look at the room from his angle: you may get a surprise. Nightlights can cast dramatic shadows which look extremely threatening: moving the light will usually remove both the shadow and the fear. However, like the adult, the child may have fears associated with his illness. Reassurance and understanding together with a cuddle are probably the most soothing ways of banishing the fears and helping him to sleep.

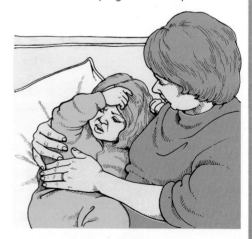

Reassuring the sick child
During illness, ordinary things in a child's room can take on a frightening character, giving rise to sleeplessness or nightmares. Reassure her that all is really as normal.

CONTROLLING TEMPERATURE
HELPING THE PATIENT TO MAINTAIN NORMAL BODY TEMPERATURE

In spite of wide variations in environmental temperature, man's body temperature stays remarkably constant: its normal range is between 36° and 37°C. The healthy body manages to achieve a balance between the heat it produces and the heat it loses. The amount of heat lost from the skin is modified by the type of food eaten and the clothing worn. Extreme external heat is counterbalanced by the heat-regulating mechanism in the brain, which cools the body down by causing increased sweating.

When the balance between heat loss and heat gain is disturbed, it is a sign that the patient has an infection or injury. When only parts of the body are affected, certain local reactions occur: this is known as inflammation. Where the whole body is involved in overcoming infection, the body temperature rises; if it goes above 37°C this is known as fever or pyrexia. If extreme cold causes the body to lose more heat than it can produce, body temperature may fall as low as 35°C: this is hypothermia.

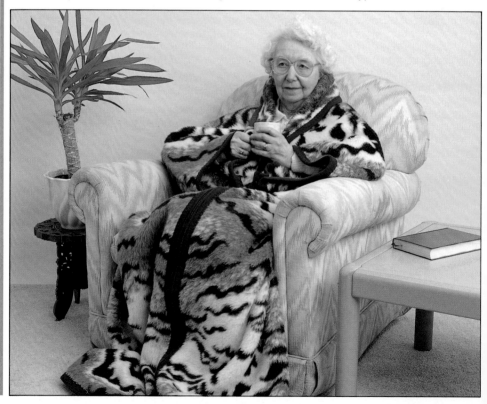

HYPOTHERMIA

The basic cause of hypothermia is a lack of external heat combined with an inability to maintain sufficient insulation. The heat loss from the body is greater than the heat produced and the body temperature falls abnormally low. Shivering occurs and the muscular activity produces heat. The heart rate increases, the peripheral blood vessels constrict and therefore the blood pressure rises. If this fails to compensate and the body temperature continues to fall, shivering is replaced by muscular rigidity, and falling pulse rate and blood pressure; consciousness is impaired and reflexes are slow. If the temperature continues to fall, coma is followed by death.

Young, fit adults exposed to extremely low temperatures can die from hypothermia if they are inadequately clothed, sheltered and fed; every year a handful of walkers and climbers die from exposure – the effects of extreme cold and inadequate clothing. In the home, it is young babies and the elderly who are chiefly at risk from hypothermia. If it is suspected, a special low reading thermometer (30–38°C) must be used.

DEALING WITH A LOW TEMPERATURE

The newborn baby
The heat-regulating mechanism in the brain of a newborn baby is not yet working efficiently, so he relies on his surroundings to maintain his temperature. It is therefore essential to make sure that a baby is kept in a warm room, possibly with additional heat at night. If the baby's room seems cold when you enter it and there is no evidence of extra heating, take a look at the baby. A chilled baby will probably have red cheeks and look healthy. This is deceptive. His

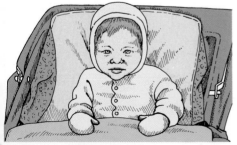

Keeping a baby's head warm
Unless the weather is very hot, a baby outdoors in her pram should have her head covered. Large amounts of heat are lost from the head, which in a baby is a very large proportion of the body.

hands and feet may be red and swollen and feel cold. His movements will be reduced and he will be too lethargic to suck.

If you come across a baby in this condition, ring for the doctor. Warm the baby gradually against your skin, perhaps by taking him into bed with you, while you wait for the help to arrive.

When you take a young baby out of doors in cold weather, warm his pram with a hot water bottle either under the mattress or at the foot of the pram, with several thicknesses of blanket between the baby and the bottle. The baby himself should be warmly clothed and covered with several light but warm layers.

The elderly patient
If when you arrive at the home of an elderly person, you find he is pale and his skin is cold to the touch, even where covered by clothing, suspect hypothermia. He may also be rather unsteady, he may be slower and more confused than usual and his speech may be slurred. His pulse will be slow and weak and his breathing slow and shallow. If you have a low-reading thermometer, take his temperature. Send immediately for the doctor. In the meantime, wrap him in

blankets and give him a hot drink to prevent him losing more heat. Do *not* use hot water bottles or electric blankets unless instructed by the doctor. If you do, the sudden heat may make the surface blood vessels dilate and draw blood away from the deep tissues and vital organs, leading to a fatal collapse caused by a sudden fall in blood pressure.

Many elderly people say they do not feel cold when in reality they cannot afford adequate heating. If this is the case, you should persuade the person to get help from the Social Security Department. At the same time encourage the wearing of shawls, cardigans, mittens, bedsocks and for both sexes some kind of hat, especially if the hair is thinning: it is surprising how much heat is lost from a bald head. Exercise will help blood circulate and tone up the muscles, even if it only consists of walking with you several times around the room. Since room temperatures always fall during the night, try to provide some kind of extra

heating: the ideal temperature is around 18°C. If there is financial need, you can suggest that the person uses one room only for living and sleeping, rather than heating two rooms or leaving a heated living room for a cold bedroom at night.

The elderly person should also be encouraged to eat a well-balanced diet; if necessary Meals on Wheels can be arranged, thus ensuring a hot meal at regular intervals (see page 67). Persuade him to take hot drinks during the day; perhaps you can leave a vacuum flask of hot fluid ready within his reach so that even if he is not very mobile he can drink frequently.

If an elderly person falls at night and is unable to summon help, his temperature may drop dangerously low and hypothermia may occur. Always suspect this if you are the one to find a fallen patient, and take steps to counteract it. Where possible make sure that someone looks in on an elderly person each morning to see that all is well.

AIDS TO WARMTH

Electric blankets and bedwarmers

There are two types of electric blanket: one goes on top of the mattress under the patient and the other covers the patient. The underblanket should never be switched on when the patient is in bed, while the overblanket is safe enough to be left on when covering the patient, because it is attached to a transformer which reduces the voltage to 20 volts. Follow the manufacturer's instructions, and make sure that

all blankets are in good condition, serviced regularly, and never allowed to get wet.

Bedwarmers are also electrically heated. They are metal containers, useful for warming a bed while the patient is up for a while. They heat a large area, especially if stood on one edge. Never leave one in bed with the patient.

Electric duvets are now available, which combine the advantages of an electric overblanket with the lightness of a duvet.

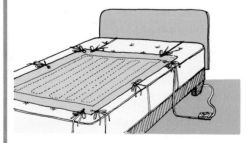

Electric underblanket
This goes on the bed between the bottom sheet and the mattress.

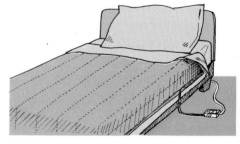

Electric overblanket
An overblanket covers the patient, over a sheet and bedclothes.

Hot water bottles

Stone and metal bottles should only be used as bedwarmers and never when a patient is in the bed. More usual now are rubber bottles, which should be completely enclosed in a thick cover before being placed in the bed, on top of the first blanket.

(Beware of bottles with a built-in cover, unless this covers the top – and many do not: an exposed stopper may burn the patient.) Never use hot water bottles or heating pads in the beds of unconscious or paralysed patients, as their normal reaction to heat has been lost and burning is likely.

FILLING A HOT WATER BOTTLE

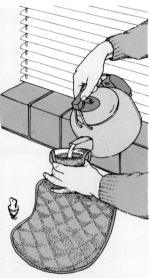

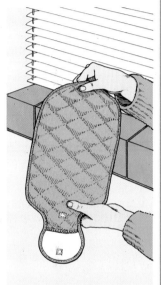

1 Lay the bottle flat on a surface and slowly fill it two-thirds full using water just off the boil. Avoid getting steam in your face.

2 Check that the washer on the stopper is not perished and expel any air in the bottle. Screw in the stopper firmly.

3 Wipe the top to remove any drops of water, and invert the bottle to make sure it is not leaking before putting it in the bed.

FEVER

You should know how to tell when a patient has a raised temperature (fever). You should also know what measures to take if it is raised. It is important to keep the temperature under control to promote recovery. If your general impression is that the patient is feverish, you can confirm this by taking the patient's temperature (see page 109). As a routine procedure, however, this is not valuable. Indeed, over the years much time has been spent in unnecessarily taking and recording the temperature, pulse and respiratory rate.

The feverish patient is hot, bright-eyed, flushed and probably sweating. He may complain of a headache, feel thirsty, have a dry mouth and foul breath. In caring for him your priorities are:

■ to make him feel cooler
■ to quench his thirst
■ to clean his mouth
■ to relieve his headache.

DEALING WITH A HIGH TEMPERATURE

There are several ways to make the patient cooler and more comfortable. A wash or bed bath (see page 44) with a change of nightclothes and bedlinen is refreshing. You can remove some blankets and give the patient a bed cradle under his coverings so that air circulates. You can also put an electric fan near the bed to move the air, as long as you do not chill the patient.

The feverish patient feels thirsty because he is sweating more than usual: sweat evaporates and cools the skin. Iced drinks are welcomed, especially sharp-flavoured ones. Frequent mouthwashes will moisten the mouth and freshen the breath.

As another result of the increased fluid loss, the patient may pass smaller quantities than usual of dark urine. If the fever lasts for more than a day or two he may also become constipated, partly because of fluid loss and partly because he is eating little. But most fevers are of short duration and small, light meals are adequate. Milky foods coat the tongue, so follow with a mouthwash.

If the patient complains of a headache, and it is severe, shade the patient's eyes from direct light and encourage him to rest quietly. A cold compress may be soothing, perhaps with a few drops of eau-de-cologne added to the water.

APPLYING A COLD COMPRESS

1 On a small tray put a bowl containing water and ice cubes. Fold a strip of linen or lint into three. Soak it in the iced water and wring it out. Hold the ends of the strip to avoid warming up the centre.

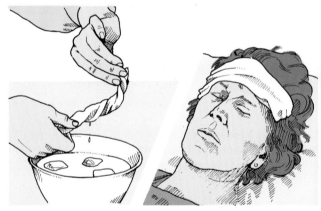

2 Apply the lint to the patient's forehead, and put a second piece in the bowl to soak. Renew as often as necessary.

FACTUAL OBSERVATIONS

To confirm your general impression of the patient's condition you may find it useful to take the patient's temperature, pulse and respiratory rate. Do not, however, write on the community nursing sister's home notes unless you are asked to. These are the notes she makes to record her nursing care, and they are used by the doctor to order treatment. She will usually leave the notes in an envelope in the same place after each visit, and you may look at them to see if there are any instructions for you. But if you have anything to report, write it on a sheet of paper and slip it into the envelope. The doctor or nurse may ask you, however, to record the temperature, pulse and respiratory rate at appropriate intervals on a temperature chart.

TAKING THE TEMPERATURE

In the mouth
This is the most usual method of temperature taking, suitable for most patients. But you should *not* take the temperature in the mouth if:

■ the patient is unconscious
■ the patient is a baby or child
■ there is injury to the mouth such as a fractured jaw, or an obvious infection

present, such as ulceration
■ the patient is likely to have a fit
■ the patient is confused.

Use a clinical thermometer, which should be stored in the case provided. If you are using it regularly, keep it dry in a small jar or in antiseptic. Before you take the temperature, rinse the thermometer in cold water and dry it with a cotton wool swab.

TAKING THE TEMPERATURE BY MOUTH

1 Shake the mercury down and place under the tongue. Ask the patient to close her lips around it, but not her teeth.

2 Wait for two minutes. Remove, wipe the bulb, read and record the temperature.

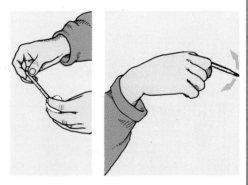

3 Shake the mercury back down into the bulb and return the thermometer to its case, or place in a jar on a tray.

Taking the temperature in the rectum
This method may be used for babies and all unconscious patients of any age. The rectal thermometer has a short bulb of the same diameter as the stem. To take the temperature, grease the bulb, gently insert it into the rectum and hold it firmly in position for two minutes. Remove it, wipe, read and record the temperature. Shake down the mercury and place in antiseptic solution. When the temperature has been taken in the rectum this should be noted on the record: rectal temperatures are a little higher than those recorded in the mouth.

Taking the temperature in the axilla
The armpit (axilla) and groin may be used to record temperature if, for instance, the patient is subject to fits or if there is injury to the mouth. When the temperature has to be taken in the armpit, this should be noted on the record: axillary temperatures are a little lower and less reliable than those recorded in the mouth. Both thermometer and skin must be dry. Lay the bulb in the armpit and fold the arm across the chest. After two minutes, remove it, wipe, read and record the temperature. Shake the mercury down and place in antiseptic.

TYPES OF THERMOMETER

Digital thermometers are battery operated with a clearly readable display. There is little doubt that the accuracy of the digital thermometer is greater than that of the clinical thermometer.

To use this type of thermometer, switch it on and place it under the tongue (or in the rectum or the axilla). Note the figures changing on the display. Wait for the buzzer to sound, or for the figures to stop flashing, depending on the type: either indicates that the peak temperature has been reached. Remove, note down the reading and switch off. Store the digital thermometer dry; it should never be immersed totally in liquid. To clean, wash just the tip with hot, soapy water. Never use the same digital thermometer for

taking oral and rectal temperatures. **Disposable thermometers** are not as accurate as conventional clinical or digital thermometers, but they are entirely safe and easy to use. They are especially suitable for taking children's temperatures. When the thermometer is placed under the tongue, the dots representing the temperature change colour. The thermometer is then discarded. **Forehead thermometers** come in the form of a heat-sensitive strip or disc, which is placed on the forehead for 15 seconds. The band or number indicating the maximum temperature changes colour. Both strip and disc are re-usable, but they are not as accurate as clinical or digital thermometers.

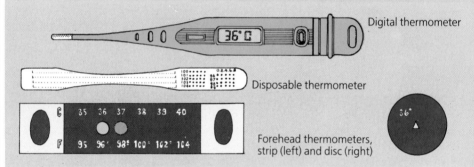

Digital thermometer

Disposable thermometer

Forehead thermometers, strip (left) and disc (right)

TAKING THE PULSE

Each time the heart beats it pumps blood into the circulation, and a wave courses along the walls of the arteries. This wave is the pulse, which can be felt in the body at any point where a large artery crosses a

bone just underneath the skin.

In a young baby the normal pulse rate goes up to 140 beats a minute, but during childhood the rate gradually falls. In the normal adult the rate is 60 to 80 beats a

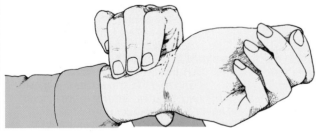

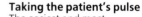

Taking the patient's pulse
The easiest and most convenient place to feel the pulse is at the wrist, just above the crease on the thumb side. Sit the patient down. Place your fingertips over the pulse and support the patient's wrist with your thumb. Count the beats for one minute. Record.

minute. There are many reasons for a rise in pulse rate: emotion, exercise, infection, shock, haemorrhage and heart disease are some of the most common. A fall in the pulse rate is more rare, but might be found in hypothermia.

As well as noting the rate, you should record the strength of the pulse – whether feeble, bounding or normal. Rhythm is also important: a normal pulse beats regularly.

It is important that you use your fingertips and not your thumb to take a pulse; your thumb has its own pulse, and you risk counting that by mistake. It is essential to use a watch or clock with a second hand for accurate counting. Practise on yourself and your friends until you feel confident to take a pulse accurately.

COUNTING THE RESPIRATORY RATE

Each respiration consists of breathing in and breathing out, so the complete rise and fall of the chest is one respiration. The normal adult breathes 16 to 18 times a minute, but a higher rate is seen in many conditions: emotion, exercise, haemorrhage and diseases of the heart and lung are among the most common causes of an increased respiratory rate.

The rate at which a person breathes can be altered at will: anyone can breathe more quickly or slowly if he wants to. Once the patient knows you are counting it becomes extremely difficult for him not to alter his respiratory rate. There is, therefore, no point in you recording it unless there is some definite information to be gained, for instance about a respiratory infection.

To count the rate accurately, the patient must be unaware of what you are doing. The best time is when he is asleep; otherwise count the rate when you are at the bedside doing something else, for example taking the pulse.

INFLAMMATION

Inflammation is the body's response to injury or localized infection. The inflamed area may be small – a boil or a stye – or it may be extensive, with large quantities of pus forming an abscess. Whatever its size, it contains a large number of micro-organisms and precautions must be taken to prevent infection spreading from any open sore. These include:

■ keeping the infected area covered
■ placing soiled dressings in a paper bag straight away and if possible burning them immediately
■ otherwise wrapping the bag in newspaper and placing it in the dustbin.

It is most important for anyone who touches the wound or the soiled dressing over an open sore to wash his or her hands thoroughly after attending to the patient, as there is a risk of micro-organisms being transferred from one person to another: this is known as cross-infection, but should not occur if proper precautions are taken.

Although infection is the major cause of inflammation, it is not the only one. After an injury such as a sprain the injured area becomes inflamed, and in diseases such as rheumatoid arthritis the affected joints are inflamed. Inflammation also follows exposure to heat – burns and sunburn – or exposure to deep X-ray or radium.

In all cases of inflammation the signs are the same: the local irritation is dealt with by an influx of extra white blood cells and the increased blood supply makes the area red, hot and swollen. The patient complains of pain and is reluctant to use or move the affected part. Apart from these local signs, if the inflamed area is large the patient may have a raised temperature (see page 107).

CARING FOR THE PATIENT WITH AN INFLAMMATION

When caring for a patient with an inflammation, the aims are:
■ to reduce the swelling
■ to relieve pain
■ to remove the infection.

If the area is large, the patient should be in bed. If not, the inflamed area should be rested. If the inflammation is in a limb, the swelling and pain can be reduced by raising the part on a pillow, or the arm can be supported in a sling (see page 125): this encourages fluid to drain away. The patient should drink at least three litres of fluid every day, to help remove impurities from the body. A mild pain-killer (analgesic) may be prescribed and, if the infection is widespread, antibiotics may be ordered. In some cases a local application of heat may be soothing and effective.

Applying local heat
The application of heat to the affected area relieves pain and may localize the infection by increasing the blood supply to the area. The treatment is often given by a physiotherapist in a specially equipped department. Radiant heat and short wave treatment are two methods of applying heat in common use in hospitals.

In the home, local heat can easily be contrived. Warmed cotton wool or an electric pad can be laid against the area. A covered hot water bottle against the ear is comforting if the patient has earache.

HOT SPOON BATHING

This is a method of applying heat to the eye if the patient has a stye.
You will need:
■ a tray
■ a wooden spoon
■ cotton wool and gauze (or linen)
■ tape for securing gauze
■ a bowl of boiling water.

Pad the bowl of the spoon with cotton wool. Cover it with a piece of gauze or linen and tie this securely around the handle. Sit the patient down and place the bowl of boiling water on a table in front of him. Let him put the spoon into the boiling water and then bring it as close to his eye as the steam permits.

Applying heat to the eye
The patient dips the spoon into the water and then brings it up as close to her eye as she can. As the water cools she will be able to bring it gradually closer to the eye, so that it almost touches the lid. She should continue until the water is no longer hot.

COMMUNICABLE DISEASES

Fever is the outcome of a generalized infection and inflammation is the result of a localized infection. There is a special group of illnesses called the communicable or infectious diseases, most of which cause fever and inflammation of the skin, glands or other organs. Serious communicable diseases are now relatively uncommon in Britain; those which do occur on the whole affect children more than adults.

All communicable diseases have certain characteristics:
■ Each illness is capable of being transmitted to others.

■ There is a specified time, known as the incubation period, between the infection of the body by the organism and the appearance of signs and symptoms.
■ In each illness every patient has the same signs and symptoms, although these may vary in the degree of severity.
■ Some communicable diseases have a characteristic skin rash.
■ Each disease lasts a certain, predictable, number of days.
■ Each disease is liable to cause complications, some of which are mild and some serious.

MODES OF INFECTION

Communicable diseases are caused by micro-organisms, which are either eaten with food or drink, breathed in from the air or which enter through a break in the skin. They are spread by people and objects. They are carried by air and dust; by infected food, water and milk; by flies and rats; by infected bedlinen, crockery and books; by

other people carrying the disease (carriers). Not everyone who is in contact with the micro-organism will contract the disease, because the body has defences against harmful organisms. It uses the white blood cells to destroy invading micro-organisms, while the lymphatic glands act as filters and remove organisms from the body.

Protect a baby from infection
A mobile baby will put to his mouth anything he comes across. Fluff on his toys may harm him; bacteria on old food certainly will.

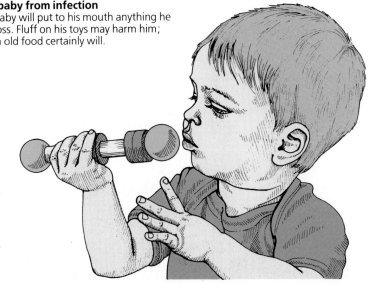

CARING FOR THE PATIENT WITH A COMMUNICABLE DISEASE

Your aims in caring for someone with a communicable disease are twofold: to provide nursing care, and to prevent the spread of infection to others.

Nursing the patient

The type of care you will give depends on the severity and seriousness of the illness. A child with a mild attack of German measles can be kept away from school for a few days and needs little nursing care. An adult with Lassa fever, on the other hand, will have to be admitted to a special isolation hospital and will require intensive medical and nursing care. In such hospitals, elaborate precautions are taken to protect the staff and control the spread of infection.

As a volunteer you have no place in an isolation hospital, but you may well be involved in nursing an infectious patient in his own home. If this is the case, it is sensible for you to take certain precautions. Eat well and avoid becoming overtired. Wear an overall to protect your clothes and wash your hands carefully after attending to the patient. Turn away from him if he coughs or sneezes when you are attending to him. He should use paper handkerchiefs, which can be put in a paper bag and burned after use, or otherwise sealed in a plastic bag and put in the dustbin.

There is little point in isolating a child with an infectious disease as most infections are caught and passed on within 48 hours. At this time symptoms may be unclear, and by the time the child develops a fever other members of the family will have already been exposed to the infection.

The patient with a communicable disease will have a raised temperature and you

The child with a raised temperature
If a child is more fretful than usual and seems off-colour, just feeling his forehead will probably establish whether he is feverish.

should nurse him as you would any patient with a fever (see page 108). If he also has an irritating rash, you can apply calamine lotion to cool and soothe the skin.

Containing infection
There are several precautions you can take to help prevent the spread of infection. Nurse the patient in a well-ventilated room where possible, with a window open except when he is being washed or treated.

Bedpans and urinals should be taken to the lavatory immediately after use and the contents flushed away. The community nursing sister will advise you if you need to take any other precautions.

Any food left on the patient's plate after he has finished should be removed and disposed of quickly. Use a fly repellent spray to keep the bedroom and lavatory free of flies and insects.

Give the patient newspapers, magazines and paperback books to read that can be burned after use. If the patient has handled a library book, seal it in a plastic bag with sticky tape and return it to the librarian with an explanatory note. Try to give a child inexpensive toys that can either be burned or washed thoroughly after he has recovered from the illness.

You must be careful not to transmit infection yourself: wash your hands after attending to the patient, after emptying a bedpan and whenever you leave the bedroom before handling anything else.

When the patient is fully recovered, strip the bed. Either send the soiled linen to the laundry or wash it in a washing machine at a very hot setting. Open the windows and air the room thoroughly.

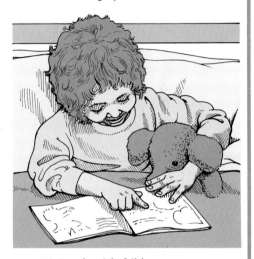

Entertaining the sick child
An undemanding picture book may absorb a sick child confined to bed. Cheap, colourful books are best: if necessary they can be disposed of once the illness is over.

IMMUNITY

Once the body has been infected by a particular disease, it can produce antibodies which give life-long immunity to that disease – few people contract chickenpox, measles or mumps more than once. There is, however, no lasting immunity against some diseases – like the common cold – so the patient has repeated attacks.

Immunity can also be acquired by immunization. A worldwide immunization policy has resulted in the eradication of smallpox; in Britain immunization has almost eliminated diphtheria and polio-myelitis, and has greatly reduced the incidence of whooping cough, measles, tetanus and tuberculosis (see page 167).

There is evidence that the number of children being immunized against these serious diseases is now falling. This may be partly the result of complacency born of ignorance – today's parents have not seen the effects of these diseases – and it may partly be fear that the vaccine used to immunize the child may be harmful. Recent publicity – about whooping cough vaccine, for instance – has led to increased concern among parents. There is always a small risk in giving any vaccine, but the risk to young babies from whooping cough is generally considered far greater than the risk of the vaccine. If you are in doubt as to what you should do, talk to your doctor.

CARING FOR A WOUND
HELPING THE PATIENT WITH AN INJURY

A wound is a break in the skin, and may be the result of an injury or an operation. Wounds need special treatment, depending on their size and severity. If they are severe enough, they may cause a raised temperature (see page 107). Any adult can cope with cuts, grazes and small burns or scalds; but, if the injury is larger, and posing some risk to the patient, professional help may be needed and the patient may have to stay in bed or in hospital for many weeks.

However large or small the injury, the aim of nursing care is the same:

■ to prevent micro-organisms entering the body and causing infection
■ to hasten healing.

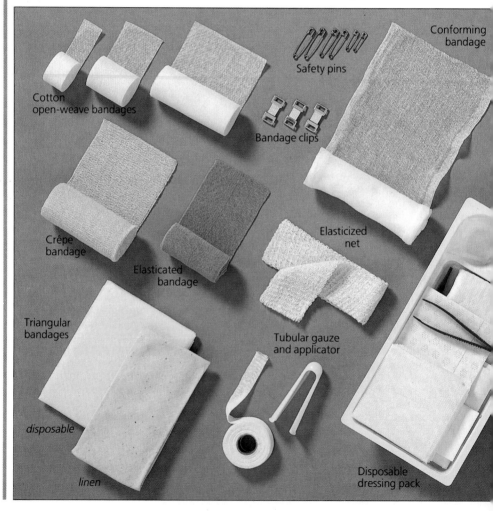

Conforming bandage

Safety pins

Cotton open-weave bandages

Bandage clips

Crêpe bandage

Elasticated bandage

Elasticized net

Triangular bandages

Tubular gauze and applicator

disposable

linen

Disposable dressing pack

116

HOW A WOUND HEALS

When any part of the body has been destroyed by disease or injured in an accident, the adjacent tissues at once begin to repair the gap. This process is known as healing. A clean cut will heal more quickly than an area where tissue has been lost, such as a burn or an abscess.

When injury occurs, the wound bleeds and the space is filled with clotting blood. White blood cells begin to destroy and remove dead and damaged tissue. Cells grow rapidly into the clotted blood and form granulation tissue. Gradually this is replaced by firm, fibrous tissue. This is known as a scar. It is often red and a little raised, but eventually contracts and shrinks into a thin white line.

Healing is influenced by many factors. Tissues require oxygen and foodstuffs – especially vitamin C – in order to repair themselves. Age is important: babies and children heal much more rapidly than the elderly. If the general health is poor from a long illness or inadequate nutrition, the substances needed for healing will be in short supply. If the patient is anaemic he will require iron, so that the blood can carry sufficient oxygen for the tissues' needs. Finally, local irritants such as a foreign body or infection will also delay healing.

The patient should therefore be well nourished and have adequate vitamin C and iron in his diet. Rest is essential. Prevention of infection is also vital.

The healing process

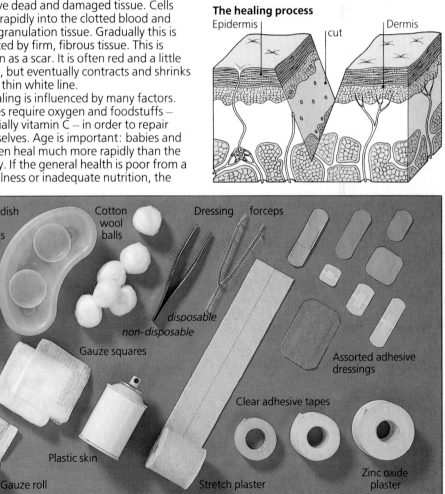

Epidermis | cut | Dermis

Kidney dish and gallipots

Cotton wool balls

Dressing forceps

disposable
non-disposable
Gauze squares

Assorted adhesive dressings

Clear adhesive tapes

Plastic skin

Gauze roll

Stretch plaster

Zinc oxide plaster

PREVENTING INFECTION

The area must be cleaned so that any dirt is washed away and the wound must be covered with a dressing. A satisfactory dressing prevents micro-organisms from entering the wound but is porous enough to allow sweat to evaporate. If the dressing is not porous, the skin becomes moist, the dressing damp, and organisms multiply.

The most efficient way of preventing infection entering a wound is to eliminate micro-organisms from everything that comes into contact with the patient. This is done in two ways:
- by sterilizing equipment
- by using a "non-touch" technique when applying dressings.

STERILIZING EQUIPMENT

Micro-organisms are destroyed by fire, by steam under pressure, by boiling, by gamma radiation or chemical disinfection. Once organisms have been destroyed, the equipment can be used with safety. It is now usual for equipment to be sterilized either at the time of manufacture or in the Central Sterile Services Department (CSSD) of a hospital.

Disposable equipment
Everyone is familiar with pre-packaged sterile dressings, which may be bought from the chemist. They are part of a range of items sterilized by the manufacturers. The equipment is sealed into plastic or paper covers and sterilized, often by exposure to gamma radiation from a nuclear reactor. Unless the package is damaged in any way, the equipment remains sterile until the seal is broken. For extra safety, many articles are wrapped in two covers.

Gauze dressings, cotton wool balls, paper towels, foil containers for lotions, instruments, syringes and catheters are all sterilized in this way. It is also possible to obtain small plastic sachets of sterile lotion.

For convenience, all the equipment and dressings needed to carry out a nursing procedure, perform a minor operation, or

dress a wound, are often packed together and sealed in a paper bag or packet. This is sterile and ready for use at any time. After use, everything should be put into a paper bag, wrapped in newspaper and put in the dustbin or burned.

Non-disposable equipment
Some items (such as glass syringes, metal or polythene jugs and bowls) are too expensive to be thrown away after use. In hospital the Central Sterile Services Department packs and sterilizes these items and delivers them to the wards and departments. After use, they are packed immediately in a paper bag, sealed and returned to the Department where they are cleaned, repacked and sterilized ready for use once more.

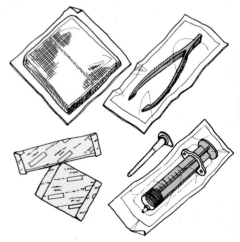

Disposable sterile equipment (right)
Many common items of nursing equipment are widely available pre-packed and sterilized. Any damage or staining indicates that an item is no longer sterile.

CHECKING PACKAGES BEFORE USE

Inspect all sterile packages before use. If dated, check that the date has not passed. Check plastic packages to make sure they are not torn; check paper packages for wetness or for any staining that might suggest they have been damaged by water at any stage. Any package that allows fluid to penetrate, is torn or has passed its expiry date, is no longer sterile and *must not be used*.

In an emergency most equipment can be adequately sterilized by immersing it in boiling water and boiling it for not less than three minutes.

PREPARING TO TREAT A WOUND

In modern hospitals a room is set aside for the treatment of wounds, but in older hospitals and in the home this is not possible. However, certain precautions should always be taken whenever a wound is dressed, to avoid contamination by micro-organisms. Avoid disturbing the air, either by draughts or excessive movement, as if dust and micro-organisms are moved they may settle on the wound. If the room needs cleaning, do this at least one hour before attending to a dressing, to allow time for the air to settle: use a vacuum cleaner if possible. Clean any trays or trolleys to be used with soap and water and check that the sterile packets are undamaged.

Avoid unnecessary talking throughout the procedure, to keep the number of micro-organisms breathed out from the nose and mouth to a minimum. Wash your hands before you start.

Which method you use to apply a dressing and how you secure it to the part will depend on the size and position of the wound and on what equipment is available.

In the home, you are likely to be attending to a small graze, cut or burn, in which case the minimum of equipment is necessary. Occasionally you may assist the doctor or community nurse with a larger dressing but in these circumstances they will provide the necessary sterile equipment. Volunteers who are helping in the Accident and Emergency Department of a hospital or in a hospital ward will have sterile packs provided, which someone will show you how to use.

There are two methods of applying a dressing to a wound: one is just a clean method, while the other involves a "non-touch" technique. There are several ways of securing the dressing, depending on the size and position of the wound (see pages 116–17 and 121–4).

SAFEGUARDS

Contamination with blood or other body fluids from a patient who has an infection in his bloodstream may be transmitted to you through cracks or abrasions on your unprotected hands.
Follow these rules:
■ Always wash your hands carefully with soap and water after attending to any patient.
■ If you suspect the patient has an infection, wear disposable gloves.
■ Mop up any spills of body fluids or drops of blood and disinfect using 1 part household bleach to 10 parts of water.
■ Place dressings and infected material in a plastic bag, seal and burn.
■ Put all needles and sharp items in a cardboard box or tin immediately after use and dispose of them as described on page 80.

Treating a small graze

The vast majority of dressings done in the home are to cover small or shallow grazes. The people most likely to suffer such grazes are children.

To dress a small graze, seat the patient and wash your hands thoroughly. Grazes often have dirt and grit embedded in them, so wash the area gently with soap and water until it is really clean. Then apply a self-adhesive dressing. Most dressings of this sort come off of on their own accord a few days later. If you want to remove it, pull it off quickly rather than picking at it; the bath is a good place to remove old plasters. If you notice any redness around the dressing, take it off and examine the graze, for redness is a sign of infection.

Grazes are often more painful than deeper wounds, because they expose an area of raw, tender skin full of sensitive nerve endings. A child who has grazed his skin needs a cuddle, plenty of attention and perhaps a sweet for bravery.

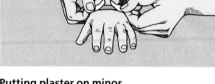

Putting plaster on minor wounds

Sit the patient down. Take the plaster out of its wrapper and peel back the protective strips to expose the gauze: do not remove the strips yet, and do not touch the gauze. Place the dressing on the wound and gently pull off the strips.

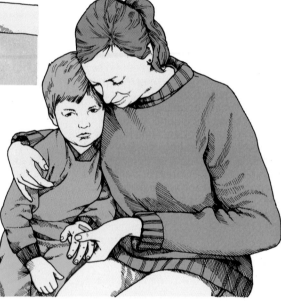

Comforting a child

A child will feel comforted if you put a plaster on his wound.

Treating a larger wound
You will need:

■ a tray
■ cotton wool swabs and mild antiseptic
■ a paper towel or square of kitchen roll
■ the appropriate dressing
■ a bandage or adhesive plaster
■ a paper bag for soiled dressings
■ a pair of scissors.

Before you begin, make the patient comfortable: seat him, or if he is in bed turn back the bedclothes, exposing him as little as possible. (If the injury is on the foot or leg, turn the bedclothes up from the foot of the bed.)

Expose the wound, removing any bandage, dressing or plaster already in place. Wash your hands thoroughly, then begin gently cleaning the wound: use cotton wool swabs dipped in antiseptic and wipe from the centre of the wound outwards. Use each swab once only, discarding them immediately after use into the paper bag. Cover the wound with a clean dressing and secure it in position with a bandage or plaster (see pages 116–17 and 121–4).

USING A "NON-TOUCH" TECHNIQUE

This is a technique which might be used by the community nursing sister, in which case you may be asked to help her. It involves handling everything that comes into contact with the patient with sterile forceps.

You will need:
- a tray or dressing trolley
- a sterile bowl for lotion
- sterile cotton wool swabs
- two sterile paper towels
- sterile gauze and wool dressings
- three or four pairs of sterile dressing forceps
- antiseptic lotion
- plaster removing solution
- a bandage or adhesive plaster
- a paper bag for soiled dressings
- a receiver for soiled instruments (if they are not disposable)
- a pair of scissors.

Note that one (or two) pairs of forceps are contaminated by the soiled dressing, and discarded immediately; then one new pair of forceps comes into contact with sterile material only, and the other comes into contact with the wound.

When you have finished, everything must be discarded into a paper bag and burned or put in the dustbin. Clear the tray away. Leave the patient comfortable.

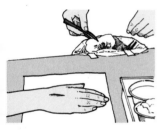 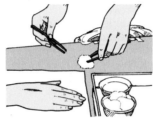 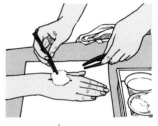

1 Close the windows and seat the patient comfortably. Wash your hands. Prepare the dressing tray. Remove the outer bandage, and discard into the paper bag. Wash your hands again. Using one or two pairs of forceps, remove the soiled dressing. Discard both dressing and forceps into a paper bag.

2 Take a fresh, sterile pair of forceps in each hand. With your left hand, pick up a cotton wool swab with the forceps and dip it into the antiseptic lotion. Transfer the swab to the forceps in your right hand, touching only the swab with the forceps. This avoids contamination of the forceps in your left hand.

3 With your right hand clean the wound from the centre outwards. Use the swab only once and discard immediately. Repeat until the wound is clean, making sure you never swap hands or forceps. Take the fresh dressing in the forceps in your left hand and transfer to those in your right. Lay it on and secure.

SECURING A DRESSING

It is essential for dressings to remain in place, so they must be carefully secured. The way to secure a particular dressing depends on what type it is.

Adhesive dressings These are small pads of gauze with a waterproof adhesive backing, which is often perforated to let moisture evaporate. They are supplied in paper or plastic containers.

Adhesive plasters Strips of adhesive plaster can be cut from a roll to secure small dressings. Waterproof plasters are especially useful for areas such as the hands.

Stretch plasters These are used to cover quite large dressings. They also give some measure of support.

Clear adhesive tapes These are used in cases of allergy or in areas where the skin is sensitive and might react to plaster, for instance around the eyes.

Plastic skin This can be sprayed on to a wound from an aerosol can. Many patients discharged from hospital have this type of dressing, which gradually flakes off.

Tubular gauze Especially useful for fingers and hands, tubular gauze makes a neat, firm bandage. It is supplied as a seamless roll, and is available in various widths to fit different parts of the body. It is applied with a special applicator. Apart from the finger size, tubular gauze is not practical for use in the home: it is expensive and a different applicator is needed for each part of the body. If thought advisable for a patient at home, the community nursing sister will supply you with the appropriate applicator and full instructions.

Elasticized net bandages Made of two-way stretch tubular mesh, these bandages are easy to apply and comfortable to wear. They are especially valuable for securing dressings to difficult places such as the head, shoulder, thigh and groin. The bandages can be cut to the required length and stretched over the dressing, and because they do not fray, holes can be cut where necessary to form a sleeve or a trouser leg. You need the correct width of bandage and a little practice to make sure of a good fit.

Roller bandages At one time, these were used extensively to secure dressings, because they provided support while restricting movement. Nowadays different methods are used, and roller bandages are applied less frequently. However, it is still useful to know how to apply one.

Roller bandages are strips of material: they can be cotton, crêpe, flannel, calico or special paper. They are five to six metres in length and their width varies depending on the part to be bandaged and the age and size of the patient.

You will need:
- a width of 2.5cm to bandage a finger
- 5cm for a hand
- 5cm for a head
- 5–6cm for an arm
- 7.5–9cm for a leg
- 10–15cm for a trunk.

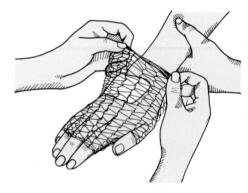

Applying an elasticized net bandage
First stretch the bandage over your hands, then place it over the dressing. Adjust the ends.

APPLYING A TUBULAR GAUZE BANDAGE

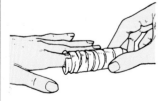

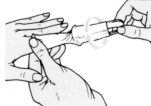

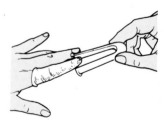

1 For a finger or thumb, cut a length of gauze two and a half times longer than the area to be covered. Push it on to the applicator. Gently push the applicator over the finger.

2 Hold the end of the gauze in position, and pull the applicator off with the other hand. Twist the applicator once or twice: no more, as you may impede the circulation.

3 Push the applicator back over the finger to its base: it will now be on the outside of the bandage. Withdraw the applicator, leaving two layers of gauze on the finger.

APPLYING A BANDAGE

Seat the patient comfortably and support the injured part. Always stand in front of the patient. Apply the bandage evenly and firmly. Too tight a bandage will restrict the patient's circulation and one that is too loose will fall off.

A wound or injury should be rested. If the patient is in bed, support the arm or leg on a pillow; if he is up support the arm in a sling (see page 125) and the leg on a stool.

Rules for bandaging
■ Hold the bandage with the roll uppermost.

■ Commence with a firm fixing turn.
■ Apply it from inside outwards and from below upwards.
■ Use a firm, even pressure for every turn.
■ With each turn cover two-thirds of the previous one.
■ Avoid covering the tips of fingers and toes, if possible.
■ Fasten off the bandage with a small safety pin or bandage clip.
■ Place a pad of cotton wool under the bandage where any two skin surfaces can rub together, for instance under the armpit. This is to prevent friction and soreness.

BANDAGING PATTERNS

SIMPLE SPIRAL

This is only suitable for use on limbs that are of roughly uniform size along the area to be bandaged, for example a forearm or a finger. Support the limb before you start.

1 With the roll uppermost and rolling it from the inside outwards, secure the end with a firm turn below the injury or dressing.

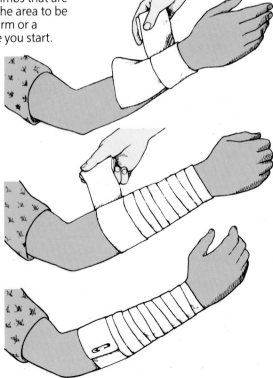

2 Work up the limb making spiral turns with the bandage. Cover two-thirds of the previous turn with the next. Keep an even pressure on the bandage.

3 When the dressing is adequately secured or the injury supported, make a straight turn at the end. Fasten with a bandage clip or safety pin.

FIGURE OF EIGHT

This pattern of bandage is suitable for awkward joints such as the ankle.

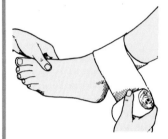 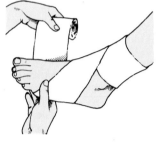 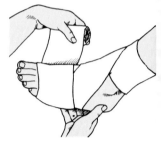

1 Support the foot before you start. Working from the inside outwards, make one straight turn around the ankle first.

2 Take the bandage across the top of the foot from the inside of the ankle to the little toe, take it under the foot and up by the toe joint.

3 Bring the bandage across the foot to the little toe and make a turn underneath to bring it up by the joint of the big toe again.

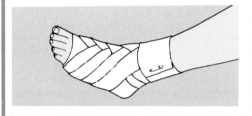

4 Take the bandage back up across the top of the foot and round behind the ankle. Continue figure-of-eight turns until the whole foot is covered. Finish with a straight turn around the ankle and secure the end. Check the patient's foot after a short delay and re-apply the bandage if the toes become cold or blue.

DIVERGENT SPICA

This pattern is a variation on the figure of eight and is used for a flexed joint, such as a knee or elbow.

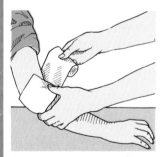 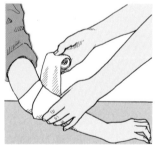 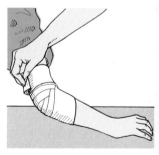

1 Support the arm so that the elbow is bent. Start at the inside of the elbow and carry the bandage around the joint to make one fixing turn.

2 Take it around the forearm, then the upper arm, working in a figure-of-eight and covering a little more than two-thirds of the previous turn.

3 Continue turns alternately below and above the elbow. Finish with a straight turn round the upper arm and secure with a safety pin or bandage clip.

APPLYING A SLING

Slings are used when it is necessary to give support and protection to an upper limb when the patient is out of bed. A sling will support the hand and arm, and is made out of a triangular bandage: you can buy one, or make one yourself out of a large square piece of linen.

Before you begin, sit the patient down comfortably and support the injured arm with the wrist and hand slightly higher than the elbow. Stand in front of the patient with a prepared triangular bandage.

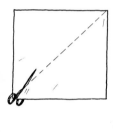

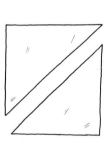

Preparing a triangular bandage
Fold a piece of linen or calico 1m square diagonally in half. Cut along the fold. This makes two bandages.

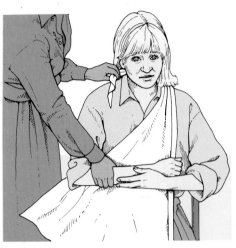

1 Hold the bandage by one short edge. Ease it into position between the patient's chest and the injured arm, with the point beyond the elbow, and the top of the long edge positioned by the far side of the patient's neck. Take the top corner round the back of the neck.

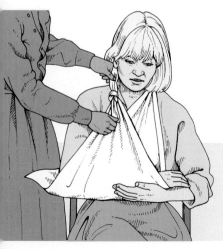

2 Carry the lower end of the bandage up and over the arm to the neck on the injured side, and tie off with a reef knot in front of the hollow above the collarbone.

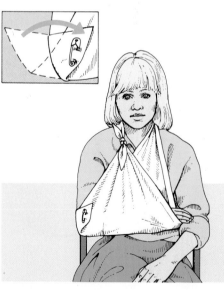

3 Bring the point forward and secure it in front of the injured elbow. If a safety pin is used, it should be secured vertically rather than horizontally.

BREATHING DIFFICULTIES

HELPING THE PATIENT TO BREATHE MORE EASILY

The beginning of a new life is measured from the moment when a baby takes its first breath. Breathing is vital to life. Because of this, breathing difficulties are always serious or, at the very least, disturbing for the patient. Nursing care in a large number of unrelated conditions may involve anticipating possible difficulties in breathing, or relieving existing ones.

It is important to understand what happens when we breathe. Adults breathe sixteen to eighteen times a minute, and the

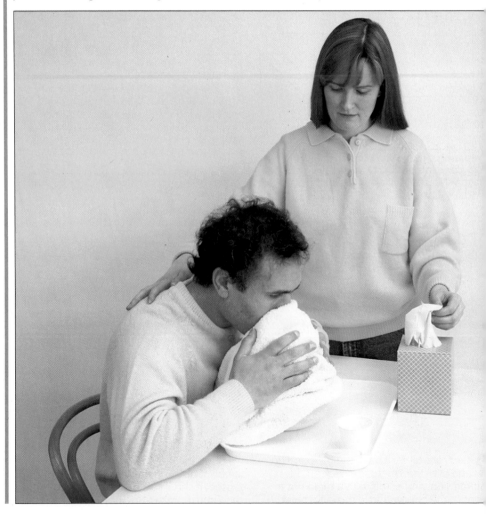

rate increases with exercise. With each breath, air is drawn in (ideally through the nose) where it is warmed and filtered by small hairs before it passes through the pharynx and larynx, down the trachea to the lungs. The trachea is stiffened with C-shaped rings of cartilage which prevent it from collapsing. It divides and sends a branch to each lung, where it divides further into smaller and smaller air tubes (bronchioles), terminating in air sacs (alveoli). The air sacs are the spongy substance of the lungs, and it is here that oxygen constantly passes into the blood and carbon dioxide is removed from it.

If anything interferes with the normal breathing process, breathing becomes difficult. Your task is to help the patient breathe more easily and you should therefore have some idea of what is causing the obstruction. All sorts of conditions may cause breathing problems: a cold may block up his nose, causing him to breathe through his mouth until his throat is sore; he may inhale a crumb or a drop of liquid, making him cough until it has been expelled; he may suffer from asthma, finding it very difficult to breathe out during an attack; or his lungs may be full of fluid, as is the case with certain categories of patients who have been confined to bed for some time.

The respiratory system

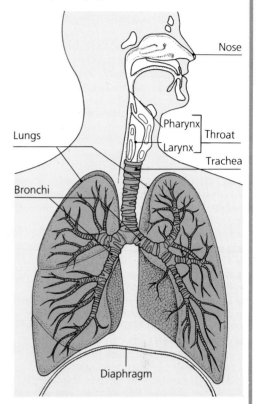

Labels: Nose, Pharynx, Throat, Larynx, Trachea, Lungs, Bronchi, Diaphragm

HELPING THE PATIENT TO BREATHE

For the patient to breathe easily, his air passages must be kept clear. This may be a straightforward matter of making sure he changes position frequently, or it may require some active care. The patient may have a cough that needs to be controlled, or the asthmatic may need his spasm relieving. You may also have to help the patient to clear a blocked nose. In every case, you should assess his general condition and decide on the amount of help he needs to breathe normally.

CLEARING A BLOCKED NOSE

If the patient's upper respiratory passages are blocked or irritated, they may be soothed and moistened with the help of steam inhalations. These are made by mixing a drug with almost boiling water (boiling water may vaporize irritant substances as well as the soothing ones), and allowing the patient to inhale the vapour.

Several different drugs may be mixed with the water depending on the patient's needs: friars' balsam is soothing and reduces inflammation in the trachea (tracheitis) and in the bronchi (bronchitis). Menthol, eucalyptus and pine help to clear the air passages by shrinking the mucus membrane lining the nose and the sinuses. Which drug you use, and in what quantity, will depend on the instructions given to you by the doctor or community nursing sister. In the absence of instructions, however, the usual dose is 5ml of friars' balsam to 600ml of water, or 1–2 crystals of menthol to 600ml of water.

To give a steam inhalation, you will need:

■ a tray
■ a large one-litre jug
■ a cover for the jug
■ a bowl in which to stand the jug
■ water just off the boil
■ the appropriate drug and a measure
■ a large towel
■ a sputum cup or plastic yoghurt pot (if required: see page 130)
■ paper handkerchiefs.

With the patient sitting upright in bed, place a bed-table or bed-tray in front of him or pull a locker or table as close to the side of the bed as you can. If the patient is in a chair, place a small table in front of him. If his nose if very sore, smear the area with petroleum jelly before starting treatment.

Pour half the water into the jug and add the drug. Add the remaining water, but do not fill the jug more than two-thirds full. Wrap the cover around the jug and place both in the bowl on the tray, with the sputum cup and paper handkerchiefs. Place in front of the patient. Help him to arrange the towel over the jug and the mouth and nose. The patient should then breathe in through his mouth and out through his nose while the steam rises (this will be for about 10 to 15 minutes). He can place the towel over his head and the inhaler like a tent; women patients, however, usually prefer to arrange the towel so that it just covers the face, as it is less likely to make their hair limp.

After the treatment, clear away and leave the patient comfortable. If he is up and about, suggest that he remains in the warm for the next half hour.

Other methods of clearing the nose can be used: sprays can be squirted into the nose or nasal drops can be given (see page 79). Always follow the instructions on the labels with care. Do not use for more than seven days without seeing your doctor.

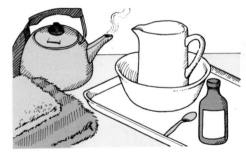

Equipment for a steam inhalation
Prepare a tray with the jug and bowl, the inhalant, the cover and the towel.

CONTROLLING THE COUGH

Coughing is a protective mechanism; it is the body's way of clearing the air passages. Some coughs are hard and dry while others are productive – that is to say, a great deal of mucus is coughed up (expectorated).

If the cough is hard and dry, the doctor may prescribe a linctus. This eases the pain and distress of coughing, which is particularly necessary at night when the patient most needs undisturbed rest. A linctus should never be diluted as the syrup-like consistency soothes the irritated passages when sipped slowly.

If there is a great deal of sputum to be coughed up, a cough mixture (expectorant) will be given to the patient to make the mucus thinner and easier to cough up.

All such medicines should be given according to the instructions for administering drugs on page 76.

RELIEVING SPECIAL PROBLEMS

Relieving asthma
The spasm that occurs in asthma is relieved by various tablets, injections and aerosol sprays prescribed for the patient by the doctor. Make sure that they are always within the patient's reach and that he has a bell near him so that he can summon you if he has an attack. Tight clothing should be avoided, especially around the neck, as during an attack an asthmatic feels as if he is being strangled. An asthmatic attack is very alarming to a child or adult, so offer positive reassurance.

Relieving hiccups
When the large muscle dividing the abdominal and chest cavities (known as the diaphragm) goes into spasm, hiccups occur. Hiccups can be extremely distressing, especially if prolonged. Sit the patient upright and try the everyday remedies: get him to hold his breath, to drink from the opposite side of a glass, or to blow up a paper bag. In most cases, one of these will work. If, however, the attack is prolonged and distressing, notify the doctor.

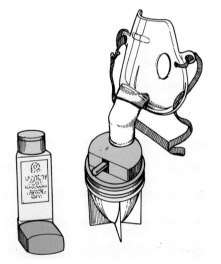

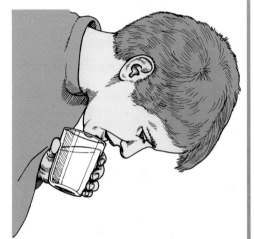

Curing hiccups
There is no infallible method of curing hiccups. However, sometimes the sheer effort of concentration needed to drink out of the opposite side of a glass is enough to relax the diaphragm and stop the hiccuping.

Drugs for asthma sufferers
Regular sufferers may have an aerosol inhaler (left) or a nebulizer (right).

RELIEVING BREATHLESSNESS

Various conditions cause breathlessness, which may be chronic or intermittent: the most common are severe diseases of the chest and heart. Before you can plan your nursing care, you should assess the patient's needs carefully. The help you give will depend on several factors: whether he is breathless all the time or only occasionally; whether breathlessness only occurs when he is walking or climbing stairs, or also when he is at rest; whether he is blue (cyanosed) or breathing more rapidly than usual. Any sudden breathlessness or change in the patient's breathing pattern should be reported to the doctor. What follows is general nursing care only.

HELPING THE BREATHLESS PATIENT

Most patients with breathing difficulties find it easier to breathe when sitting upright. A backrest and pillows will help while a board or pillow to support the feet will stop the patient slipping down the bed. This is important: if a patient with severe heart disease slips down the bed, he may, especially at night, have an attack which so closely resembles an asthmatic attack that it is known as cardiac asthma. Sometimes these patients are given a special suppository before being settled down to sleep (see pages 87–8). The drug is absorbed through the rectum into the bloodstream and reduces the spasm in the bronchioles.

Occasionally at home the breathless patient is nursed sitting up in an armchair. In these circumstances you must see that he changes his position regularly, and that his feet and legs are kept warm. Keep the room well ventilated at all times. Avoid giving dry foods, which will cause coughing; but do give frequent, small, light meals that will tempt the appetite but not overload the stomach and so put pressure on the diaphragm. If his air passages are dry and inflamed, a steam inhalation (see pages 127–8) may bring relief. If he is cyanosed, oxygen may be prescribed.

The doctor will probably ask you to observe several specific things about the breathless patient: his colour, respiratory rate and sputum.

Colour

If the patient has an infection he may be flushed. If there is insufficient oxygen in his blood he is cyanosed: his skin will have a bluish tinge, especially around the nose, mouth and the lobes of the ears. Note if the blueness is improving or not as a result of treatment, or if it is worse at any particular time of the day.

Respiratory rate

Difficulty in breathing will alter the patient's respiration and it may be necessary to count the respiratory rate (see page 111), so that the doctor can assess the effect of his treatment. This may have to be done regularly over a period of time.

Sputum

Sputum is fluid coughed up from the lungs. It varies in quantity, colour and type. Patients who produce small quantities of sputum may spit into paper handkerchiefs. Any patient with a productive cough should have a waxed carton into which to spit: if a carton is unobtainable, a plastic cream or yoghurt pot with a lid is an acceptable substitute. At least once a day the paper handkerchiefs or carton should be placed in a plastic or paper bag and burned, or wrapped carefully in newspaper and put in the dustbin.

Remember that sputum may contain bacteria and could be a source of infection. Sputum containers should always be kept covered and should be handled carefully, especially at the time of disposal.

The doctor may ask for a specimen of sputum to be saved. If it is for laboratory examination he will supply the appropriate carton. Your duty is to make sure that the carton is clearly labelled with the patient's name, address, the date, and the nature of the content.

GIVING OXYGEN

Frequently in hospital and sometimes at home a patient may be given oxygen to assist his breathing. Oxygen is supplied in a black and white cylinder. In the home a small size is used, but in hospitals cylinders are stored in a bank away from the ward and the gas is conveyed to the patient along pipes set into the wall. If an atomizer is used, it may be connected to a small oxygen cylinder by the bedside.

The oxygen is under considerable pressure inside the cylinder. Because of this, a special valve is fitted, called a reducing valve, which prevents the gas coming out too quickly. The amount of oxygen the patient is receiving is measured in litres per minute by a flow meter. The amount of oxygen in the cylinder is measured by a pressure gauge, indicating full, half full or quarter full.

In hospital oxygen may be given through nasal catheters by face mask, or by placing the patient in an oxygen tent. At home oxygen is most usually given by face mask.

Always observe safety precautions when in the presence of oxygen (see overleaf).

An oxygen cylinder

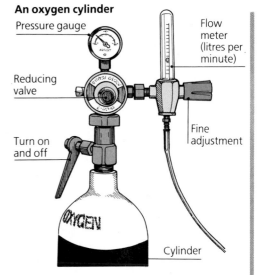

Pressure gauge

Flow meter (litres per minute)

Reducing valve

Turn on and off

Fine adjustment

Cylinder

TURNING ON THE OXYGEN

Check that the cylinder is an oxygen cylinder. Read the pressure gauge to make sure the cylinder contains oxygen. Connect the breathing apparatus to the supply, but do not place it over the patient's face yet. Open the cylinder with the key and adjust the rate of flow according to instructions (it is measured in litres per minute). Check that the oxygen is flowing by holding the mask near your cheek, then arrange it comfortably for the patient. Record the amount given in litres per minute.

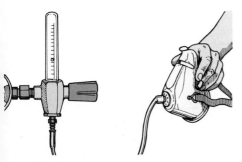

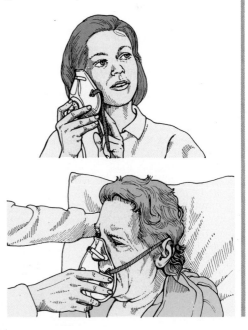

1 Check that the cylinder contains oxygen. Connect the apparatus to the supply.

2 **Above right:** Open the cylinder and adjust the rate of flow. Hold the mask to your cheek to check that oxygen is flowing.

3 **Right:** Place the mask over the patient's face so that it fits snugly and comfortably over his nose and mouth.

Portable oxygen apparatus

Many patients with chronic lung, chest or heart complaints are helped by being able to breathe oxygen when climbing stairs or moving about. In these cases the family doctor will refer the patient to a consultant, who can prescribe the most suitable apparatus which the hospital will then lend to the patient and maintain.

There are several makes of portable oxygen cylinder available, each supplied with a shoulder strap and carrying bag. They weigh between 2.5 and 5kg each and hold from 100 to 500 litres of oxygen. The patient is also supplied with a gauge and a face mask.

Portable cylinders can be filled from an ordinary oxygen cylinder, with the help of a special recharging adaptor. No special skill is needed and the procedure takes about twelve minutes. Many chemists now operate a while-you-wait refill service, in which case the doctor may prescribe an extra cylinder.

It is possible to buy more sophisticated or elegant pieces of portable oxygen equipment than those available through the National Health Service, but they are generally very expensive.

Using a portable cylinder

A portable oxygen cylinder may allow a breathless patient to enjoy a greater degree of mobility than would otherwise be possible.

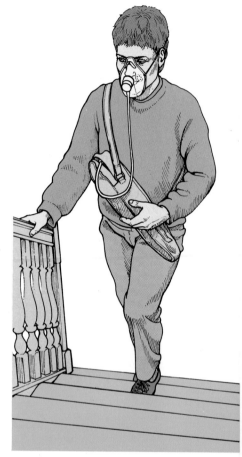

DANGERS OF OXYGEN

Whether oxygen is used at home or in an institution, the dangers are the same. No naked light or spark (such as from a mechanical toy) must be allowed to come anywhere near oxygen: fire spreads with frightening rapidity in the presence of this gas. Smoking is strictly forbidden for the same reason: a glowing cigarette will burst into flame.

Grease or oil should not be used on the valve or flow meter, nor should these be touched with greasy hands. Grease and oil may ignite spontaneously in the presence of oxygen, causing an explosion.

Oxygen cylinders, whether full or empty, can be dangerous if played with by children or if stored for a long time.

If you remember these things when dealing with oxygen, you should be safe:
■ no sparks
■ no smoking
■ no grease.

CARING FOR A TRACHEOSTOMY

An increasing number of patients breathe through an artificial opening in the neck called a tracheostomy. You should be aware of the reasons for this if you are to care for the patient adequately.

The operation is carried out when there is an obstruction to breathing like a growth in the voice box (larynx) or, more rarely, because of severe flame or caustic burns. A hole is opened up in the patient's neck and a tube inserted through the hole into the trachea. As a temporary measure, unconscious patients being nursed in an intensive care unit or patients with severe respiratory problems may be artificially ventilated through a tracheostomy. In these cases, when the patient is better the tube is removed and the opening heals. In other cases the tube may be permanent.

Should you be helping to care for a patient who has had a tracheostomy, as part of your daily care you may be asked to look after his tube. This consists of an outer tube, which you must not remove, and an inner, which can be taken out for cleaning. This is particularly important if he has a chest infection, as mucus can clog up the tube and obstruct his breathing. The community nursing sister will demonstrate the procedure, and in an emergency ask the patient or a relative how the tube is normally cleaned and follow their instructions. In the absence of any instructions, rinse the tube either under running water or in bicarbonate of soda solution (one 5ml spoonful of bicarbonate of soda to 600ml of water). Rinse it well before returning it to the patient for use.

If the patient's voice box (larynx) has been removed he will be unable to talk. Some people are taught by a speech therapist to manipulate air belched from the stomach to produce speech (see page 136). If the voice box is still there, a little valve in the tracheostomy inner tube closes when the patient wishes to speak.

Tracheostomy

A tracheostomy is an easy operation, which may be performed under either a general or a local anaesthetic. A tube is inserted to open an air passage between the trachea and the front of the neck when the throat or larynx is blocked or damaged. The tracheostomy may be temporary or permanent.

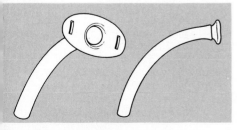

The tracheostomy tube
The tube comes in two parts: the outer is secured by tapes and stays in position all the time; it should only be removed by a doctor. The inner can be removed for regular cleaning.

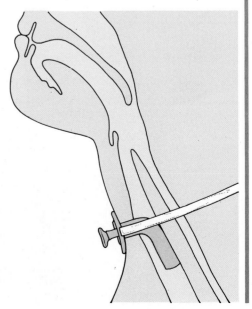

COMMUNICATION
HELPING THE PATIENT TO COMMUNICATE HIS NEEDS EFFECTIVELY

Communication is an essential social process. People need to communicate: to express their anxieties and their emotions, to make known their wants, and to go about their daily lives. As a volunteer you should be sensitive to all the ways in which a patient may try to communicate, whether these are verbal or non-verbal. In certain illnesses where the patient has difficulties in making his needs known, what little verbal communication there is may be especially important from a practical point of view, while non-verbal communication forms a valuable basis for many observations.

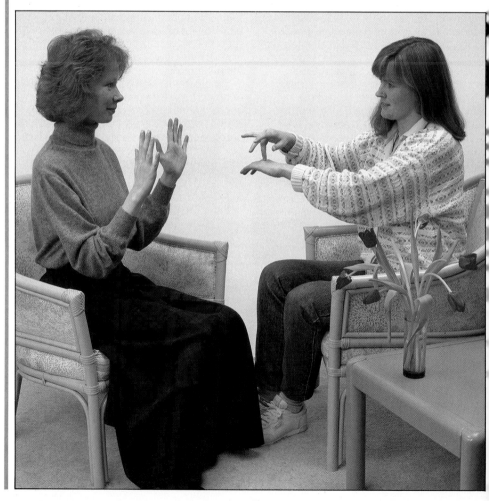

NON-VERBAL COMMUNICATION

Animals exist entirely without the spoken word. They make friends, find mates, rear young, establish their territories and co-operate in groups using only expressions, posture, gesture, smell, and noises. Much human communication is also non-verbal. A person's facial expression reveals if he is happy or angry. A sagging posture suggests weariness, dejection or unhappiness. The outstretched arms of the mother promise love and security. A handshake is a mark of introduction and acceptance; in some business circles it acts as a bond. Movements of the head may denote agreement or disapproval. From earliest childhood we are taught to recognize these signs and many others. Learning to be sensitive to them is part of learning to live in society.

It is not difficult to apply your knowledge of people in general to the patient. When entering a patient's room you observe his face: he may look tense, totally blank, or have a face screwed up with pain. Caught unobserved, the weary or dejected person slumps in the bed or chair, the depressed person tends to huddle in a corner, and the person with a headache lies with his face turned away from the light or with his hands covering his eyes. The person with abdominal pain tends to lie on his side and draw up his legs. The frightened person grips your hand or arm, the frustrated child bangs his head against the side of his cot and the agitated elderly person mutters to himself. These signs of the patient's feelings are all relatively obvious; the better you know an individual patient, the more easily you will come to recognize non-verbal signals far more subtle than these. Understanding the unspoken feelings of your patient, however they are expressed, will help you to care for him better.

VERBAL COMMUNICATION

Verbal communication is fully as important as non-verbal. If you cannot understand another person because of a speech impediment or the inability to speak his language, you cannot exchange ideas or share experiences. Communication is reduced to exaggerated gestures and mime. It is like shopping abroad when you do not speak the language, and can be a very depressing experience for people of all ages.

When English is not the patient's mother tongue, there are many sources of help available to the volunteer. Local authorities and some voluntary organizations often produce a range of multi-lingual leaflets to help with language difficulties, and the numbers of interpreters willing to lend their services are increasing. The volunteer should always try to use adults as interpreters, as a child's vocabulary is often not wide enough to communicate adequately.

Verbal communication can also become a problem if disease or damage interfere with the normal speech processes.

COMMUNICATION PROBLEMS

One of the main difficulties experienced by voluntary workers is uncertainty about how to approach the patient, whether his disability is physical or emotional. This can be overcome by obtaining help and advice from the community nursing sister, health visitor or specialist social worker. Be sensitive to the needs of the patient and anticipate his wants. Try to understand how his condition is affecting his ability to communicate. Be patient and give him the time and opportunity to express his wants and feelings. If you have no other time to set aside, often during a bed bath or other similar procedure there is the opportunity and the time to encourage the patient to talk.

Always address yourself directly to the patient, even if he cannot answer or he is handicapped. People have the habit of talking as if the patient were not present. They address his companion to ask "Well, how is he today?" Imagine how frustrated you would be if you were the patient. Even if he cannot respond, include him in the conversation. Talk about your leisure activities, or any subject that will give him interest and pleasure. This is especially important if the patient is confined to one room.

THE PATIENT WHO CANNOT TALK

The patient may be unable to talk (aphasic) as the result of a stroke. His hearing is not affected and he knows what he wants, but he cannot tell you. Some patients can speak, but due to brain damage or disorder they are incapable of saying the right word; after much effort, they come out with a word that is quite inappropriate. This causes further distress.

Quite literally these patients have to be taught to speak again. This requires patience on your part, and perseverance on the part of the patient. A speech therapist will assess the patient and commence treatment, but clearly cannot be with him all the time, so there is a lot of scope for relatives, friends and volunteers to help. In the early stages picture cards can help a patient to express practical needs that he cannot otherwise communicate to you: show him a selection of picture cards, perhaps made up from pictures from magazines, and he can then point to the bedpan or glass of water that he needs.

Another group of patients deprived of speech are those who have had their voice box (larynx) removed (see also page 133). Some of these patients are eventually taught to speak again, by modifying the sound produced by belching air from the stomach, but it is a long and difficult process. However successful the result, the patient's speech can never sound like a normal voice. Give encouragement and support to these patients, so that they are motivated towards speech. This group can often communicate by writing down their needs, so have a pencil always to hand.

THE DEAF PATIENT

The deaf patient's inability to hear makes it hard for him to communicate. If, as is common among the elderly, hearing fails gradually, the patient often doesn't realize he is becoming deaf and accuses other people of mumbling. Soon he begins to feel isolated and rejected and may even become suspicious and feel that people are talking and laughing about him, when in fact they are just taking part in an ordinary conversation. A hearing aid may help, and you can help the patient by finding out about the various types of aid now available, and encouraging him to wear it. But do remember that a hearing aid will magnify *all* sounds, including background noise, and may not help the patient in all circumstances. Be sensitive to this, particularly when the patient is in large groups of people. Plenty of non-verbal signs and a specialist to teach lip-reading may be as helpful to some patients as a hearing aid.

A little thought in the early stages of deafness can serve to minimize the sense of isolation. Never turn your back on a deaf person while talking to him. Try to use the lower tones of your voice range as these are more readily heard. Include the person in your smiles and gestures when possible. Because deafness often leads to a very restricted social life there is scope for much welfare work among the deaf. It is a field in which the voluntary organizations offer a great deal of help.

THE BLIND PATIENT

The blind patient can talk and can hear, but non-verbal communication is largely inaccessible to him – you cannot hear a smile or an outstretched hand. Blindness may result from injury, it may accompany another disease or it may come as part of the ageing process. Once the initial shock – which can be very considerable – wears off, the patient has to adapt to a new way of life. His hearing and sense of touch develop, he may learn braille and other new skills.

Some patients adapt readily and others do not. Ageing often brings a gradual loss of sight, allowing time for some adaptations to occur during the partially sighted period. This group of patients needs understanding and support: hearing may be failing at the same time as sight, while simultaneously patients are often becoming less active and mobile, and you may be able to help the patient come to terms with a gradual deterioration in his faculties.

DEAFNESS AND BLINDNESS IN CHILDHOOD

The deaf child
Deafness is virtually impossible to diagnose in the newborn baby, who does not react to sounds in a predictable way. A deaf baby under six months old will make babbling noises just like a normal baby. But it is essential to diagnose deafness early in order to make use of every scrap of hearing the child may have: it is by imitation of sounds heard that the child learns to talk and so communicate with others. Doctors and health visitors working in child health clinics therefore pay special attention to hearing tests. Even a six-month-old baby can be fitted with a hearing aid and so learn to interpret sounds.

Deaf children attend special schools where no effort is spared to teach them the art of communication. Hearing aids, micro-phones, lip reading, mime, sign language and machines which reproduce sound as patterns of light are all used to this end.

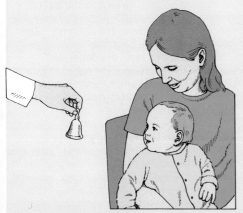

Testing a baby's hearing
Deafness needs to be diagnosed early, so any mother worried that her young baby cannot hear should request a simple hearing test.

The blind child
Total blindness at birth is not common, but a number of children have sight defects serious enough to necessitate special attention at school. The totally blind infant usually goes to a residential nursery school, where he is trained to move about independently. His education continues at a special school with emphasis on teaching by sound and the use of braille for reading.

THE NON-ENGLISH SPEAKING PATIENT

Patients whose first language is not English may have difficulty in communicating unrelated to any physical impairment. Often they have the additional disadvantage of being unfamiliar with British culture and the British way of life. Women in particular often become severely depressed with no contacts outside their own family; relatives may need to be persuaded to allow them to visit a doctor. Cultural influence must be respected: for instance, some Moslem women are reluctant to undress, particularly if they are to be examined by a male doctor, so do what you can to have them attended by a woman doctor and arrange for relatives to be present as well, if that will help.

Try to communicate with these patients somehow, whether it be through another member of the family or an interpreter. Try also to arrange for these patients to meet and talk with other people who speak their language, and to join in social activities with them. The more frequently you attend to someone in this position, the more easily you will understand the patient's needs, and the easier the patient will find it to transmit emotions and fears. As a practical measure, there is much bi-lingual material available that may help you get the answers you need to perform your nursing duties.

THE CONFUSED PATIENT

Temporary confusion may occur if a patient has a high temperature or is suffering from mental illness; in the latter case the confusion may arise as a result of the illness itself or of the treatment given. Most confused patients, however, belong to the older age groups. A confused patient may not know where he is, what day of the week it is or what he wants. He may wander about in a dazed way and do potentially dangerous things. Always make sure the doctor knows if a patient is confused as all types of patient may benefit from some medical treatment.

Confusion associated with infection
When the patient has an infection, confusion may arise from the toxic state and from the dehydration caused by the raised temperature. This will generally be only temporary: replacement of fluid and reduction of temperature bring speedy improvement.

Confusion in the elderly
The elderly often become confused when they are moved to different surroundings – to hospital, for instance, to a nursing home or to a relative's home. Not uncommonly in these circumstances they cling to a particular nurse or volunteer, insisting that she is their daughter, niece or long-lost friend. Something in the appearance or manner of the individual probably triggers off a memory and the association is made. The confusion is often lessened if the number of people involved in the patient's general care is reduced; adding vitamin B to the diet and improving the patient's general health may also be beneficial.

If the patient's sight or hearing are impaired the problem is increased. Much patience is needed among those caring for this group and repeated explanations of the simplest things may be needed.

Confusion in the mentally ill
Confusion from mental illness may arise as a result of the illness itself or of the treatment given. If you want to communicate with the mentally ill, it is not just a matter of establishing contact with the patient, but also the difficulty of overcoming barriers within yourself. People are often over-anxious and even frightened of mental illness, and do not know how or where to begin to help the patient with his difficulties.

HELPING THE MENTALLY ILL

Volunteers who are caring for the mentally ill often ask: "What should I say?" There is no magic formula, no easy answer, but with care and thought it is unlikely that anything you do or say will be harmful to the patient. If in doubt, try listening rather than talking.

Listening is often of great value. Many patients are able to unburden themselves of great misery simply by talking to a sympathetic listener who is not too busy to spend some time with them. Sit quietly, give the patient your undivided attention and you may find that you only need to smile or nod and he will be encouraged to continue. If he does not talk, just sit with him in a companionable silence. This is very comforting and is often appreciated, as the patient feels he matters to someone.

Just as the patient's spiritual adviser brings help and comfort in physical illness, he may also be of help in a mental illness. If the patient wishes it, inform the relevant person and give him the opportunity to visit. Both the patient and his family may benefit. You may also benefit: his knowledge of the patient, his family, and their cultural and religious customs may prove very useful.

The patient in the community
The patient who is being cared for in the community needs the support of his family, employer and friends. They must accept him as he is, realizing that the behaviour which seems odd or irrational to them is quite rational to him. All he says and does will be affected in some way by his illness.

The patient who has been in hospital
If the patient's condition required his admission to hospital, his subsequent return home is often effected gradually. First he goes home for weekends and then, as he improves, for longer periods, until his final discharge. Once home he may still require help and support, so he and his family will be visited regularly either by some of the team who cared for him in hospital or their community counterparts.

Sometimes the transition from hospital to home is too difficult and the patient may go first into a special hostel, a halfway house. From the hostel he goes to work, visits his family and friends, but has expert support when he needs it. When his self-confidence has returned he can resume life at home.

The majority of patients spend less than six weeks in hospital, but a return to full health takes longer than this. The majority are cured quite quickly; some take longer, but only a few are incurable.

Group therapy for the mentally ill
Patients suffering from some kinds of mental illness are encouraged to participate in group therapy sessions, under the leadership of a professional health worker. Sharing their thoughts and feelings with other patients often helps them to overcome their problems.

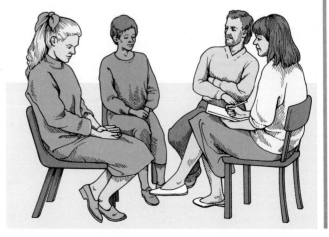

RECOVERY AND REHABILITATION
HELPING THE PATIENT TOWARDS COMPLETE RECOVERY

Pressure on National Health Service beds means that patients are now discharged from hospital as early as possible into the care of the family practitioner and the community nursing sister. As a volunteer you may be asked to help care for such patients, and to help them towards recovery.

You may also be caring for day patients in the home: these include patients who regularly attend hospital for treatment, daily or less often for short periods; and patients who attend a centre for the whole day from Monday to Friday. It will help you to know what is happening to them during this time.

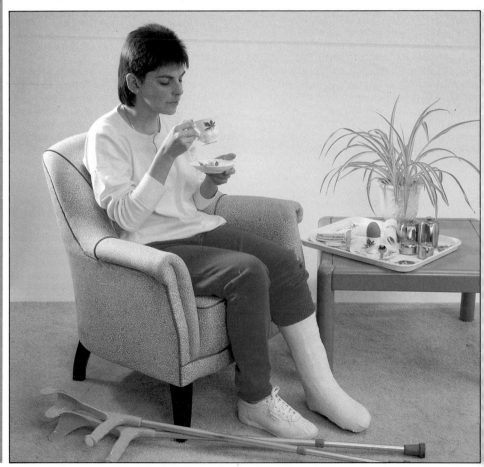

PATIENTS NEWLY DISCHARGED FROM HOSPITAL

When a patient is discharged from hospital into the home, you will need information on a number of points in order to assess his condition and estimate how much and what sort of care he needs.

- How much activity may he undertake?
- How much rest should he have?
- Are there medicines to be given?
- Are there arrangements for dressings to be changed or stitches removed?
- Has he an outpatient appointment?
- When may he return to work?

It is a great temptation for a patient to think that, once he is home, he is absolutely fit and can do anything. The housewife particularly tends to come home and take over the household duties at once. In fact, the newly discharged patient tires easily, as he is always much weaker than he suspected when pottering round the ward. In spite of his eagerness to get home, he is often restless and depressed, finding it hard to settle down. He may be missing the security of the hospital ward. Tolerance and understanding help the patient through this phase of recovery.

All convalescent patients, irrespective of age, should be encouraged to rest for at least an hour every afternoon, preferably on the bed where they can really relax. To allow for enough rest, domestic help may be needed. If members of the family cannot provide this, private help or a home help should be suggested. The Social Services Department provide a home help service where it is needed, with the patient paying according to his income.

All patients need to take exercise, and the doctor will guide you about the amount. Plenty of fluids and an interesting diet appetizingly served will also promote recovery. The patient may need help with shopping and the provision of meals. Neighbours, the home help and young people in voluntary organizations are often willing to help with the shopping, while the Meals on Wheels service may be able to provide a midday meal (see page 67).

Your nursing care and the advice you give will obviously depend on the patient's condition. The patient recovering from an abdominal operation, for instance, should avoid lifting and carrying. Certain patients have special needs. These may be practical, psychological or both. If the patient has had an operation such as a mastectomy, for instance, she will need practical help in choosing a suitable prosthesis but above all she will be in need of psychological support. Any operation that involves removal of a part of the body destroys self-image and is emotionally distressing. You will need to be sensitive to the feelings of these patients.

If a treatment such as a dressing or injection is required, the community nursing sister will visit. She will tell the family if there is any equipment she would like provided for her use. If a patient is being discharged from hospital at a weekend or bank holiday, it is essential to make sure that the hospital provides an adequate number of dressings for the patient's use until a prescription can be obtained from the doctor and dispensed by the chemist.

THE CONVALESCENT CHILD

A child needs special understanding after a stay in hospital, even if one or both parents have been able to stay with him for most of the time. The unfamiliarity of hospital combines with any pain or uncomfortable

procedures to disturb the child and make him feel insecure. For a while after his return home, especially if the stay has been long, the child may behave as if he were younger than his years. This is known as regressive behaviour and it may take many forms: the exploring toddler may become clinging, shy and more dependent on his mother than usual, the child competent at feeding himself may revert to bottles, and the child dry for over a year may start wetting his pants. If the family and all those caring for the child offer love, security and understanding, the child will gradually regain his normal level of development.

The convalescent child
A child may show regressive behaviour after a period of illness. Be patient if she wants you to do things for her, and cheer her up with toys and unusual drinks.

THE NEW MOTHER

The mother with a new baby is usually tired and often anxious. A demanding baby is causing broken nights and generally disturbing the household; and often the most tiring aspect of the newborn baby's behaviour is its unpredictability. Until a few weeks have passed and the baby has settled into a pattern, the mother can never be sure what the baby is going to do. She cannot be immediately sure why he is crying, whether he is still hungry or if he is sleeping enough.

In these circumstances the new mother should be offered as much help and support as possible. She may become tense and anxious, but if she can be encouraged to remain calm she will communicate a relaxed feeling to her baby, who will respond by settling more quickly. The community or home midwife usually visits the mother and the baby at home for ten days after the birth, with the health visitor taking over on the eleventh day. If there is anxiety about the mother – particularly if she seems depressed or the baby is not well – contact the midwife, health visitor or family doctor as soon as possible.

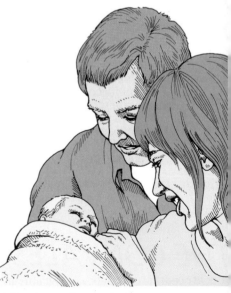

Adjusting to the new baby
Both mother and father have to get to know their new baby, and need plenty of time to relax and adjust to the change in their way of life.

DAY PATIENTS

People who attend hospitals or centres as day patients may do so for a variety of different reasons. Patients attending hospital may be receiving continuous daily treatment or they may be attending regularly, but intermittently, for a specific course of therapy. Patients attending a centre may also receive treatment, but this is likely to be combined with social activities. Some centres provide only a social service.

Patients receiving outpatient care or regular treatments of radio- or physiotherapy often need transport. Generally the hospital will arrange this for them.

DAY SURGERY

Nowadays patients are often admitted for surgical procedure and discharged the same day. As with any operation, it is essential to see the hospital's instructions about the last meal and last drink before admission are followed and any medicines by way of preparation are taken at the correct time. The family will be advised when to telephone or return to the hospital to collect the patient, and will be given instructions as to after care and follow-up visits to hospital. During the day make preparations for the patient's return, remembering that many will wish to retire to bed as soon as they reach home. Most will appreciate a light meal. If pain-relieving tablets have been supplied by the hospital, you will need to see these are taken as instructed.

DAY TREATMENTS AT HOSPITALS

Radiotherapy
This consists of directing at the affected part of the body special X-rays that destroy diseased or unwanted scar tissue while leaving the surrounding tissue undamaged. Precautions are taken so that the radiation cannot penetrate any area other than that needing treatment. Patients often attend the hospital as day patients. A course of treatment may last from four to six weeks and leave the patient very weak. Nausea is not uncommon and the patient is often reluctant to eat.

The skin over the treatment area may become red and sore, particularly if it is an area where sweating and friction occur, such as the armpit or the skin under the breast. The patient will be given very detailed instructions on how to care for the area and these must be followed exactly, as many soaps, powders and creams in common use only aggravate the condition.

As treatment continues, weakness and tiredness increase and vomiting and diarrhoea may occur. Morale is low. The patient – already apprehensive because of his disease – feels the treatment is having no effect. Encouragement and support are vital at this stage. As a volunteer, you may well be familiar with the patient's symptoms: they are the result of radiation and are less severe manifestations of those seen in radiation sickness caused by nuclear activity. The difference is that the patient is receiving *controlled* doses of radiation. When the treatment stops, the symptoms will disappear, so you can reassure him that his discomfort will pass.

An alternative treatment involves the intravenous use of chemical substances which destroy abnormal cells without damaging normal tissue. The patient will be treated as an inpatient, and will need a tremendous amount of help and support.

Physiotherapy

This is given for many muscular and joint conditions. It is also used to re-educate limbs that have been immobilized after surgery or fracture, and limbs weakened after a stroke. Exercises are often taught as part of the treatment and the patient may need encouragement to persevere. Physiotherapy may also involve teaching breathing exercises before and after an operation.

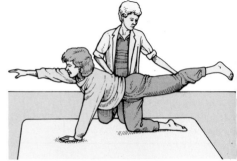

Giving physiotherapy (above)
A patient needing physiotherapy will be treated by a trained therapist, who may prescribe a course of regular exercises for the patient.

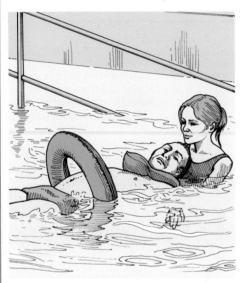

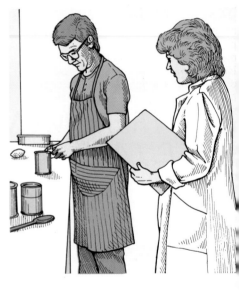

Hydrotherapy (above)
The patient is immersed in warm water so that exercising becomes easier and less painful.

Occupational therapy (right)
This is used to rehabilitate patients who have suffered a stroke or similar handicap.

ATTENDANCE AT DAY CENTRES

Day centres have been established in many areas. Handicapped and elderly patients are collected by ambulance or voluntary transport in the morning and taken to a centre (which may or may not be in a hospital) where they spend the day. Here there may be facilities for physiotherapy, hydrotherapy and occupational therapy. The patients are also given a well-balanced midday meal. Social activities are often included, so the patients are kept occupied all day; they return home in the evening.

The voluntary organizations are actively concerned in the work of many of the day centres. They may fetch patients and take them home, organize social activities, and offer nursing care if necessary, such as bathing or feeding patients. In many cases, without the help of volunteers it would be impossible to staff day centres adequately.

OUTPATIENTS

Whereas day patients usually attend hospital for post-operative treatment, outpatients most commonly attend for pre-operative investigations.

It is impossible to mention all the reasons why someone may have to attend the out-patient department, but a little knowledge about some of the more common may prove useful, and may help you to give the patient the support he needs.

Plaster of Paris

Patients with a fractured limb, particularly an upper limb, have plaster of Paris applied and are then sent home. While the plaster is drying, avoid direct heat and support the part comfortably on a pillow. There is a danger that the injured limb may swell inside the plaster and cause constriction, so if the patient feels increasing pain in the limbs, if the fingers or toes look blue, swollen or feel cold, it is advisable to take him back to the hospital.

Dilatation and curettage (D & C)

A dilatation and curettage is a scraping of the womb (uterus), done to examine the lining of the womb as an investigative or diagnostic procedure in a gynaecological examination: it may be carried out after the patient has suffered excessive or irregular bleeding. Afterwards there is likely to be a heavier blood loss than during a menstrual period, but after 24 hours this should begin to decrease. Encourage the patient to take it easy until the bleeding has stopped.

Barium X-ray

Barium is a substance which shows up on an X-ray film. It is given by mouth to outline the stomach when there is a gastric complaint, and X-rays are taken at specified intervals to follow the progress of the barium through the small and large intestine and discover any abnormality. Barium may also be given as an enema.

A day or two before the investigation, the patient may be given tablets to take. These are usually to empty the rectum and reduce the gas in the intestine. He will also be given full instructions on his diet in the days preceding the investigation, and may have to fast. Because barium is white, the patient will pass white stools for a short while afterwards, and he may also be constipated.

Gastroscopy

Gastroscopy also investigates conditions of the stomach. A flexible tube is passed through the mouth into the stomach. With the help of a light and a series of mirrors, the doctor is able to look at the stomach lining. Patients often complain of a sore throat and have difficulty in swallowing for a day or two after gastroscopy.

Cystoscopy

This is a similar type of investigation, but in this case the tube is passed into the bladder. It is common to experience discomfort when passing urine for 24 hours after the investigation. Blood may also be passed. Encourage the patient to drink plenty of fluids as this helps to prevent infection and makes it easier to pass urine.

Scans

While an X-ray takes a single two-dimensional picture, a scan gives a detailed three-dimensional picture on a monitor. **Ultra-sound scans** use sound waves to give information about the liver, kidney, thyroid and pregnant uterus. The procedure is safe and painless. The whole area is smeared with jelly and the probe rubbed gently and systematically over the skin. The image of the organ appears on the monitor. **Whole body scanners** are large, expensive machines which move a narrow beam of X-ray in a pre-arranged pattern. The patient should be warned that he will be placed partially or completely inside a tunnel. The procedure is noisy and takes anything from 5 to 30 minutes. The patient will be alone in the room, although always in voice contact with the operator.

RECREATIONAL ACTIVITIES
HELPING THE PATIENT TO MAKE GOOD USE OF HIS TIME

Recreation means exactly what it says: recreation. It covers any activity that is found to be refreshing and renewing. Patients need it as much as anybody else, but many find it almost impossible to think up stimulating ways to pass the time, or to arrange activities for themselves.

As a volunteer you have a very special part to play in helping with recreational activities. You may just be concerned with the needs of one patient in the home; on the other hand, many volunteers visit hospitals and homes for the elderly or disabled to talk with patients, write their letters and play games with them. Others are asked to help with group activities such as sing-songs and outings. Their involvement is invaluable not only for the patients but also for those nurses and helpers who staff the homes and hospitals.

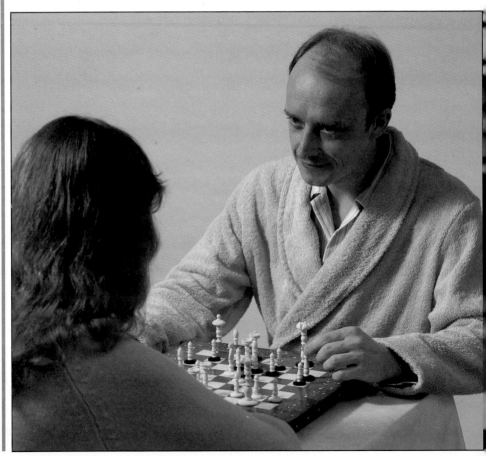

PLANNING RECREATION

Recreation must be carefully planned and designed to suit the patient's particular need. The better you know an individual, the more accurately you will be able to tailor your suggestions to his needs, but there are several general points to consider.

Much will depend on the patient's age and sex as well as his health. Most important, what are his interests and what facilities are available for him to pursue them? If illness has imposed limitations – mental or physical – on his ability to pursue his interests, these should be considered. In certain cases it may be possible to combine recreation with the patient's rehabilitation: something as easy as going for gentle walks, for example, may give the patient pleasure and help him to regain fitness.

STAGES OF ILLNESS

The amount of time during the day that the patient has to spend on recreation and the enthusiasm he displays will partly depend on the stage of his illness.

At the height of his illness the patient will tire easily and his powers of concentration may be reduced. Even at this stage planning some recreation into his day will help to counteract the debility and depression felt during and after an illness.

Radio and television demand no physical activity and can be very useful in amusing someone who is ill or elderly. Many housebound people find comfort in participating in broadcast religious services; others find it pleasurable to watch sport. Every effort should be made on your part to avoid meals or nursing care during the patient's favourite programmes. Make sure that the television or radio is properly adjusted and that it is neither too quiet nor too loud. If the patient cannot reach the controls, be available to switch off or over when he tires. If the patient loves music and a record- or cassette-player is available, put on his favourite records; if he is in hospital inquire if the hospital broadcasts a request programme on its own wavelength.

Patients who can hardly move because of weakness or paralysis can derive a great deal of pleasure from bird life. Hang a nut basket or piece of fat near the patient's window and keep the bird table stocked with bread and seeds. An extraordinary number and variety of birds will be attracted to it. These patients may also take pleasure in watching a few fish in a bowl, or even just having a new picture to look at on the wall; these can often be borrowed from a local picture library.

Once the patient is capable of greater concentration, he may want to start reading again. The short articles of a magazine or newspaper may be easier for him to absorb at first than a full-length book. Or consult the local librarian and try to get hold of some art or travel books with more pictures than text. These are often of interest to the patient, especially if you can chat together about places you have visited. The patient may, of course, have his own ideas about what he wants to read, which you must respect. If his sight is poor, try to borrow large print books from the library.

Remember that all large books are heavy and the patient may need to prop them up against a bed-table or a pillow.

There are specially recorded readings known as talking books now readily available; the totally blind may be supplied with a machine to play them. Some areas even have a weekly or monthly talking newspaper with all the local news.

Many women, and some men, may be interested in knitting, crochet or needle-work. During illness they might be diverted by learning a craft they haven't done before – macramé, for example. A walk round a good handicraft shop will keep you up to date with new ideas.

147

Some patients may be attracted by jigsaw or crossword puzzles; others may be stimulated to draw or paint. The patient will probably enjoy a game of cards, chess or "Scrabble" if you or a friend can be persuaded to drop in for an hour or so.

People in hospital eagerly await the trolley shop to buy writing paper, soap and other small necessities. The housebound can derive the same pleasure from shopping by post. This allows them to choose things for themselves and to plan small surprises for other members of the family at birthdays and Christmas.

ACTIVITIES FOR THE CONVALESCENT

As convalescence progresses and the patient begins to be up and about, a walk in the garden to see the flowers and the vegetables creates an interest and a sense of achievement. The keen gardener will enjoy gardening programmes on radio and television and will gladly read gardening books, but even more, he will appreciate a vase of flowers from his own garden or an indoor plant to tend. The elderly or handicapped may be able to continue gardening if there is a raised flower-bed or if they are supplied with a suitable kneeler – some types have handles to help the user lower himself down and then get up again afterwards. Light tools will help someone with weak limbs and hands.

After a long illness a walk as far as the pillar-box or round the block is a great boost to the patient's morale. A short car ride can also be very pleasant, especially if the driver uses a little imagination, and can take the patient into the countryside.

If patients are severely handicapped or need activities to get stiff limbs moving again, the occupational therapist will give help and advice. You only have to think of the Olympic Games for the Disabled to see what can be achieved in spite of difficulties. At the same time you should be realistic: just as most ordinary people are unlikely to compete in the Olympics, most of your patients will not reach Olympic standard either. The important thing, in this as in all recreational activities, is to capture the patient's interest and relieve the tedium of illness for a short period. If you are successful in this aim, all the energy you put into planning interesting and varied activities for him will be well worthwhile.

Pursuing interests after illness
Practical help may be necessary to enable someone keen on gardening to keep up their interest after an illness, or when old age makes limbs weak and stiff. A much higher raised bed may even enable a wheelchair patient to garden.

PLANNING ACTIVITIES FOR CHILDREN

Children pose a special problem. When they are very ill they are not interested in much except perhaps a favourite toy to cuddle or a story. But as soon as a child begins to feel better he is easily bored and needs constant attention. Keeping him occupied becomes difficult, particularly if he is not well enough to play with brothers and sisters or friends.

A convalescent child confined to bed will not stay quiet beneath the bedclothes. Because his movements in and on the bed will disturb the bedclothes, he will stay much warmer if he is dressed.

If you are buying toys, give the child one or two small ones every day rather than a big toy expected to engross him for the length of his illness. This way every day will bring him something new and relieve the monotony – especially important in sickness when you cannot expect the child to concentrate for long.

If you are giving the child puzzles or games, start with an easy one and progress to something more suited to his age as he gets better: a sick child is likely to give up in frustration and misery if he cannot do a puzzle, whereas the same child when well would have the determination to carry on trying until he is successful. Lego and jigsaw puzzles are very popular with sick children.

Small doses of radio and television may be relaxing for a child confined to bed. Make sure that you are at hand to turn the set on or off and to change channels if the child is not allowed out of bed.

Drawing and painting are much enjoyed by ill or convalescent children. Even quite small children can be successfully occupied for long periods in colouring picture books. If you are encouraging messy activities, do make sure that both the child and the bed are protected: an old sheet is very useful for this. If the child is painting put all his equipment on a tray and give him a non-spill paint pot, or a pot with very little water.

Try to make a game out of nursing care and tell stories while you are bathing the child or carrying out any treatments. Above all, remember that ill children need even more love and attention than usual. Take time to give the child a special cuddle, especially at the end of the day when he may be restless, hot and tired. Sit him on your knee to read a story: this is one of the best ways to soothe a restless child to sleep.

If the child's illness or convalescence is going to be prolonged, the parent or volunteer can seek outside help with recreational activities. Youth organizations such as the Girl Guides and the Boy Scouts may run activities for the housebound, and the Red Cross Juniors and the St John Cadets will visit to play games with the child. Encourage the child to participate in competitions run for children by television programmes such as "Blue Peter". Finally, in cases where the child will be housebound over a very long period, a peripatetic teacher may be necessary.

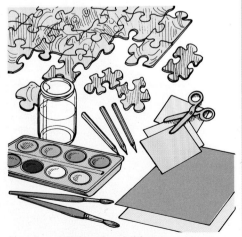

Creative activities for children
Jigsaws, a paintbox, pencils and coloured paper to cut up will all amuse a convalescent child.

LEARNING AND RE-LEARNING
HELPING THE PATIENT TO OVERCOME DISABILITIES AND MASTER NEW SKILLS

A baby at birth knows nothing about the world. To develop normally he must learn. The only way he can learn is by taking an interest in his surroundings. For this reason every healthy baby is born curious.

Curiosity is an important factor in child development. Without it the infant would not begin to explore his world: feeling, tasting and touching all the things around him, trying to find out more about them. As he grows he begins to crawl or shuffle about and eventually he walks. His new mobility enables him to make further discoveries. When he becomes able to use and understand language, he is well on the way to making sense of the world.

Every mother watches her child pass through these stages towards independence with delight and some anxiety. The young child has no sense of danger and risks injuring himself. He must be watched constantly, yet he must be allowed to be adventurous. Exploring and finding out are vital to his development.

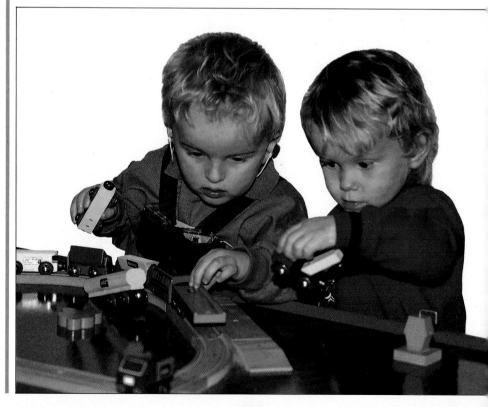

DIFFICULTIES WITH LEARNING

If his basic needs for food, exercise, fresh air and shelter are met and if he is surrounded by love and affection, the healthy child develops normally. Sometimes, however, mental or physical handicap interferes with the process of development. Although handicapped children are usually still curious, their ability to learn is in many cases impaired to some degree.

Handicap may vary from a minor disorder of function to some major disability which can never be completely overcome. The child born deaf or blind, for instance, has clear and possibly permanent obstacles to learning at the same rate as other children. But where handicap is the result of illness or injury, the child may regain his previous rate of learning in time. Whatever the circumstances, the aim of care is the same: to encourage the child to develop and learn as fully as possible, using whatever means may be available or appropriate; and by so doing allow the child to live as full a life as possible while safeguarding his self-respect and developing his independence.

Some children fail to progress in their development because of a mental handicap. Many such children seem curious but are not able to learn normally; their mental age is far below their actual age in years.

Mentally handicapped children are often loving and affectionate, but their presence in a family can impose a great emotional strain. Families in this position should call on the support and advice of professional workers, so that they can be taught how best to help their child, themselves and their families, and also be helped to build up reserves of love and patience.

For these special children every step in the learning process is hard won, and for the parent or volunteer the pace may seem very slow. The degree of handicap will govern the child's rate of learning, but even the severely handicapped child can usually master simple skills: he may eventually be able to feed and dress himself and carry out simple, repetitive tasks. However limited his potential, he must be helped to develop it to the full.

TOYS AND PLAY

All children learn through play and the tools of play – toys. Where there is handicap the selection of toys can be an integral aid to a child's development. A toy must match the mental age and ability of the child: if it is too simple it quickly becomes boring, if too difficult it causes frustration.

Toy libraries
There are some 1,000 toy libraries in the country. These not only provide a wide selection of toys suitable for different types of handicap, but also give help and support to the families of the children. Many toy libraries are run by volunteers, who advise on the most suitable toys for any one child, but there are often professional workers such as teachers and specialist health

visitors also on hand. Parents of handicapped children often feel isolated and set apart, but in the informal surroundings of a toy library it is easy for families to meet and give mutual support and understanding. Both parents and children get the opportunity to experiment with a wider selection of toys and play equipment than is normally available in the home, and the library may even create or adapt a toy especially to meet the needs of a particular child.

Babies and young children who have not yet reached the stage of making eye contact or of reaching out and handling objects can be helped by toys that make them look and touch, and so experience pleasure. A textile block, each side covered in a fabric of a different colour and texture, develops

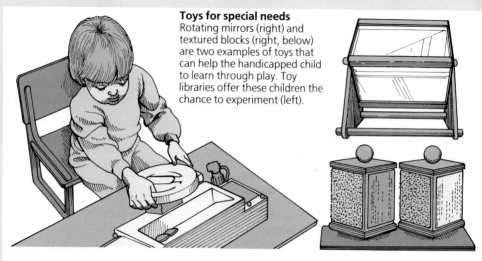

Toys for special needs
Rotating mirrors (right) and textured blocks (right, below) are two examples of toys that can help the handicapped child to learn through play. Toy libraries offer these children the chance to experiment (left).

recognition; these textures are also particularly useful for teaching the blind. Rotating mirrors which catch the light and reflect objects attract attention, and also help the visually handicapped child by maximizing the light available. Suspending objects of different shapes, colours and textures on a rail makes them easy to reach, while their dangling movements attract attention and their colours and textures stimulate the child. Children with poor hand control need toys that are firmly fixed with suction pads; those with limited movement need toys that are easy to reach. Poor coordination and manual dexterity can be improved with a series of toys of gradually increasing intricacy, with each one needing finer movements than the last. Toy libraries can also offer battery-operated toys with delicate pressure switches to children with severe weakness: often these are the only toys suitable for them. For all these children, the toy library provides the pleasure of the visit, the excitement of choosing the toy, and the fun of being with other children while they are there.

Children with Down's syndrome
Cared for lovingly, Down's syndrome children will derive great and obvious enjoyment from life's simplest pleasures.

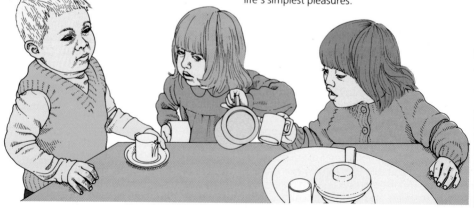

THE NEED TO RE-LEARN

In certain circumstances following an illness or an accident, an adult may have to re-learn many things. Just as natural curiosity in a child should be encouraged, in an adult it may have to be re-awakened, so that he may discover what he can do and gain enough confidence to extend himself further still. The patient who has had a stroke, for example, may have to learn to speak again, to feed himself with only one hand and chew his food with a part of his face which he cannot control. He may have to learn to walk with a paralysed leg and struggle to re-learn many simple skills he mastered as a young child.

The man who has lost an arm in an accident not only has to master the skills of everyday living, but may have to be retrained at his old job or learn to do a new one. The patient with spinal damage must learn to propel a wheelchair, re-learn the skills of driving with hand controls and adapt his daily living to wheelchair height. These are just some examples of circumstances that might make re-learning necessary.

To be successful in cases of severe physical handicap, re-education requires a team approach. The detailed planning is for the expert, but each professional worker and volunteer contributes his own special skills. The patient's family and his friends can all help in giving the care. In some cases progress is slow, while too much physical activity is damaging. You should be aware of this, and stay in close contact with the experts, so that you can consult with them before giving any care.

Resources for re-learning for the individual at home are wide-ranging. Television further education, available to anyone with a television or a radio, might be one option, another could be a corres-pondence course, which will probably require a greater level of commitment on the part of the patient. Computers and word processors also have a valuable role to play in helping some patients adapt to changed circumstances.

Retirement and old age

When the day of retirement comes it brings a loss of friends and a change in status. Income is often severely reduced. Unless they have a wide range of interests, retired people risk finding themselves lonely and bored. Because of this, it is worthwhile planning activities for retirement in some detail beforehand. People who have devoted time to thinking about how they are going to fill their days often come to find retirement a period of great fulfilment, when at last they are able to indulge in all the pursuits they did not have time to try when they were working.

Many people turn to their garden or take up golf. Others find satisfaction in the abundance of day and evening classes run by the local education authority (where senior citizens are often entitled to pay reduced fees). Such classes provide com-panionship, interest and the opportunity to learn something new and possibly make new friends. Television further education and correspondence courses may also offer intellectual stimulation.

As the years pass, however, even the most contented and fulfilled people usually find that they have to modify or re-learn skills. The normal ageing process causes the eyes to dim, hearing to lose its clarity, and people to become generally slower. Bones are brittle and break more easily, while mobility may also be affected. The sense of smell is less acute, so that smoke from a house fire or escaping gas, for instance, may go unnoticed. All or some of these gradually encroaching disabilities may eventually cause the patient to need nursing care and regular attention.

THE PATIENT WHO IS DYING
HELPING THE PATIENT TO A PEACEFUL AND DIGNIFIED DEATH

Caring for the dying is no easy task. It calls for the exercise of technical skill supported by compassion and imagination. When approached for the first time, it is often very frightening. But it can also bring deep satisfaction to those providing the care, in spite of the demands made on time, physical strength and patience.

Death comes in many forms: sometimes so suddenly that no care is possible; sometimes unexpectedly during an acute illness; more often as the expected end of a long and sometimes painful illness. Many patients in the last category may come to know or suspect that they are dying and

they may wish to be cared for in their own homes. While relatives feel they should agree to this, they are often anxious that they may not be able to cope and give the patient the care and support that he needs. The problems involved should therefore be listed and faced so that those providing the care can appreciate what is required.

If you are caring for someone who is dying you should be prepared to:
■ cope with feelings and fears about death, both your own and the patient's
■ make the patient comfortable
■ recognize the signs of approaching death
■ know what to do when death comes.

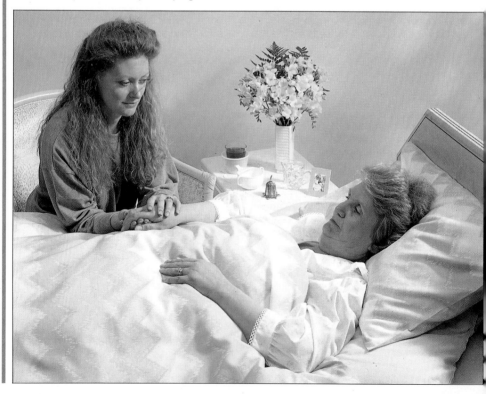

FEELINGS AND FEARS ABOUT DEATH

When a patient has been ill for some weeks and it becomes apparent that his general condition is deteriorating, he tires quickly, cannot make the effort he used to and often loses weight.

At this stage the question arises as to what the patient should be told about his illness. There is no easy answer. Much depends on the patient himself. He may know that he is dying and he may not need to ask anyone for the truth. He may ask someone just to seek confirmation of what he already knows. On the other hand, he may ask the newest, least experienced person involved in his care, "Am I going to get better?" or "Am I dying?", knowing that because of her inexperience and lack of knowledge she cannot give him the answer he does not want to hear.

Many people hesitate to talk about death. This is, perhaps, because it is the common experience we all face and yet one of which we have a limited knowledge. But at some time in our lives we all experience grief and loss. It may be the loss of a toy, a friendship, a home or a loved one; it may be the loss of a limb. As we grow older more of our friends die and we come to realize our own mortality. Grief is the reaction to our loss and the process by which we inwardly accept the reality of an event that has already occurred. It is the process by which we fill the gap in our lives after a large part of our world has been lost.

Stages of grief

Just as all those surrounding the patient pass through stages of grief, so does the patient who has learned he is dying. If we understand these stages we can cope more easily with our own feelings and, most important of all, we can better anticipate and meet the needs of the patient.

For the patient the first stage comes immediately after he has been told or has realized that he is dying. He suffers shock and disbelief: "this cannot be happpening to me; the diagnosis must be wrong; the doctor does not know everything." It is the same reaction sometimes seen in parents who refuse to admit that their child is backward or deformed. The shock may be accompanied by physical signs: fainting, pallor, nausea, gastric upsets, rapid pulse or even restlessness and confusion. Sometimes the patient may cry.

This initial reaction is often gradually replaced by an awareness of the truth as the reality begins to penetrate the patient's consciousness. He feels sad, hopeless and helpless. He may become angry and blame himself or others. Whatever you do will be wrong. If you want to bath him, he will wish to rest. If you leave him to rest he will say that you are neglecting him. His food will be too hot or too cold and never what he fancies. His medicines and treatments will always be given at the wrong time. He will not want to see his visitors but if they do not come to visit that will also be wrong.

Why is he angry? In effect he is saying: "It is all right for you; you are well, free and able to do what you want; I cannot and will never be able to do so again." He may start to bargain: "If only I can live another six months, I will . . ."; he may become very depressed, withdrawing into himself and not wanting to talk. You may even find him crying quietly. The way you can best help him at this stage is to give him time to grieve. Sit quietly with him and let him talk if he wishes to do so.

This is the point when the patient may derive most help from his spiritual adviser. The dying patient not only has emotional and physical needs but spiritual needs. Many patients find their religious beliefs all-important in their effort to gain the strength and courage to face their own death with dignity.

The third stage of grief is the acceptance of the inevitable. This final stage brings peace and a sense of well-being. The patient will seem more content and may even try to comfort those around him. He may begin to sort out his affairs and a solicitor may be of help.

Your task is to help the patient through these stages and to relieve his loneliness, depression and fears. Most dying patients have three main fears: these are fear of pain, fear of loneliness and fear of the moment of death.

Fear of pain is very common. To help the patient it is important to see that he is kept comfortable and that he receives his medicines on time. The doctor should be told immediately if the prescribed pain-killing drugs are proving inadequate. Fear of loneliness and of dying alone are also very real fears. Most people die when someone is in the room with them, almost as if they hold on to life until they can die in the presence of another human being. Reassure the patient that he will not be left by himself at any time.

MAKING THE PATIENT COMFORTABLE

As well as helping the patient to cope with his fears and worries, you must also care for his physical well-being and comfort. Your aim is to make his last days as happy and relaxed as possible, so that last memories may be pleasant ones.

The dying person has the same physical needs as any other patient. He must be kept clean, comfortable and free from pain. For as long as he is able he should continue to get out of bed, particularly to visit the lavatory or to use the commode. Movement of this kind reduces the risk of pressure sores (see page 29) and gives the patient a little interest and variety.

When the patient becomes too ill to get out of bed his position must be changed every two hours. If he becomes incontinent his skin should be washed and dried carefully and a protective barrier cream applied. An incontinence pad or Kylie sheet may be useful (see page 92). The patient must be helped with his toilet (see pages 83–4) and you should assess the degree of help he requires at any time. Mouth care will be necessary once he is unable to clean his own teeth and if he has dentures you will have to attend to them (see page 47).

The patient's appetite will be failing, so you should offer small appetizing meals of food that he likes. It is essential that he takes adequate fluids; small frequent drinks are more easily tolerated than large ones.

Try and avoid a rigid timetable: be prepared to give him a drink or something to eat during the night if he is awake and hungry or thirsty. Vomiting can sometimes be troublesome (see page 69). Constipation may also be a problem, but this can be avoided by the planned use of suppositories (see pages 87–8).

Many dying patients are not in pain, but those who are need a pain-relieving drug. Such drugs are called analgesics and they range from paracetamol to morphine. The particular drug and the dosage will be determined by the doctor and your task is to ensure that it is given regularly and at the right time. The doctor should be informed if the drugs fail to control the pain or if the patient is no longer comfortable between doses. There is, however, a delicate balance between keeping a patient pain-free and alert. If his last days are to be happy this balance must be achieved.

A Buddhist patient may not wish to have analgesics as Buddhists regard unclouded consciousness as crucial to the finest death. He may, however, be helped by quietness in which to meditate.

If the patient is restless and fails to sleep, other drugs may be prescribed.

The relatives also need help at this time. There is a great deal of physical and emotional strain. See that they eat, and take regular spells away from the bedside. Extra help may be needed so they can have uninterrupted nights of sleep, knowing that someone will call them if the patient's condition deteriorates. The local authority's night sitter service or the Marie Curie Foundation may be of help here. Macmillan nurses can advise on pain relief for cancer patients.

THE SIGNS OF APPROACHING DEATH

The patient grows weaker and sleeps more often. He does not wish to eat or drink. The power of movement and his reflexes are lost; tight bedclothes may bother him so they should be loose and light. You should check frequently to make sure that he has not become incontinent. As his circulation fails, his fingers, toes and nose become blue or mottled. His skin feels cold and clammy and he sweats, regardless of the room temperature. This is because the body temperature is rising. Most dying patients are not conscious of being cold; in fact they tend to be restless because they are hot. This fact often needs explaining to those close to the patient.

The patient will probably turn his head towards the light. As sight and hearing fail he only sees what is near and only hears words spoken clearly. For this reason do not draw the curtains or talk in whispers. As his sensations diminish he no longer feels a light touch, only pressure. This is the time to hold his hand firmly. His breathing will become laboured and noisy. He may become drowsy, go into a very deep sleep or coma, or he may remain quite conscious until the end.

It is difficult to determine how long this period will last, but it is the time when relatives wish to be at the patient's bedside. Seat them comfortably and encourage them to hold the patient's hand and talk quietly to him, whether he is responding or not. Make sure they leave the bedside at intervals to have a meal or a drink and to have a rest. The physical and emotional strain on the relatives during the last days or hours of a patient's life is enormous and it is at this time that the volunteer may be able to give both invaluable practical help and sympathetic support.

CARING FOR THE PATIENT AFTER DEATH

Once breathing has ceased, close the patient's eyelids and leave the relatives with him for a few minutes. Note the time of death. See the family doctor is informed.

When you return to the patient, remove the pillows from the bed, straighten the body gently and lay it flat. If the patient normally wore dentures and they are not in his mouth, clean them and put them in. If there are dressings, colostomy, ileostomy or urinary drainage bags, replace these with clean ones. Cover the patient with a clean sheet and leave him until the undertaker comes. He will attend to everything else. It is a matter of personal preference whether the face is covered or not. Tidy the bedroom and remove all the medicines and nursing equipment. If there are flowers, place a vaseful on the bedside table. Once all is tidy the relatives may like to be left alone with the patient for a while.

After the undertaker has removed the patient, strip the bed, air the mattress and pillows and open the windows.

Different religious beliefs
It is important to remember that certain religions require specific ceremonies at the

time of death. Try and find out about them before the patient dies so as to avoid confusion and distress for the relatives.

Jewish and Moslem patients may not be cremated and people who have to touch them after death should wear gloves. Sikhs and Buddhists are cremated and may otherwise be cared for as Christian patients. Hindus like to die at home and often on the floor, to be near mother earth, and this can usually be arranged. They do not require any special care after death.

HELPING THE RELATIVES

If the relatives are present when the patient dies, leave them with him for a few moments before gently leading them away. Once the patient has been attended to and the room tidied they may be taken back to the bedside if they wish. Find out if there is anyone they would like telephoned.

When death occurs in a hospital, relatives are usually taken to sister's office and given a cup of tea. When death occurs at home you should stay with them until a friend or another relative has arrived. Initially they may be shocked and unresponsive, however much the death was expected. Presently they may cry or begin to talk, recalling incidents and reliving the past. Sit quietly by them and listen. A silent presence is often very comforting.

Practical help

A great deal of helpful information is given to the family by the undertaker. He will want to know if any jewellery, such as a wedding ring, is to remain on the patient; if not it should be removed before he leaves.

In hospital a record is made of the patient's valuables and other property. These are then taken to some administrative office in the hospital from which the relatives collect them. A note is kept of any jewellery left on the patient and usually of whether any dentures are in the mouth.

The doctor in charge of the patient certifies death and issues the certificate to the relatives. The death certificate must be taken to the Registrar of Births, Marriages and Deaths. The final funeral arrangements can then be made.

If the doctor has not seen the patient before death or if there are any unusual or suspicious circumstances, he will report the death to the coroner or appropriate authority. The coroner will then decide whether a certificate can be issued or if a post-mortem examination is necessary. The coroner may conduct an inquest into the death; if he does, the death certificate will be withheld until it has taken place.

Many people have insurance policies especially to cover funeral costs. Most families are entitled to a death grant. It may also help them to know that undertakers vary considerably in their charges. Financial affairs should be dealt with by the family; a family solicitor can be most helpful. The local social security office will be willing to give advice about which forms should be completed for pensions and allowances.

Helping the family after a sudden death

The volunteer may be asked to help when there has been a sudden death. It may follow an accident or heart attack or some major tragedy like a motorway pile-up, or an aircraft or ferry disaster. At such times the relatives and friends are suffering from emotional shock, there has been no preparation for death, they said goodbye to a healthy son or husband in the morning never to see them alive again. The stages of grief crowd upon each other and the relative is confused, angry and desolate, they cannot accept what has happened.

The best way to help is by just being there. Listen to what the relative has to say, and don't shy away from talking about the dead person if that is what they want. Make sure they have at least a drink and try to persuade them to eat a little. Give the family any practical help that you can, such as making telephone calls, taking messages or answering the door.

AFTER THE FUNERAL

Once the death occurs there is much to arrange and relatives and friends rally to give support. It is after the funeral that the relatives start to feel lost and lonely. It matters little whether this was a sudden or long expected death. They long to talk about the dead person and remember the happy times. Too often at this point friends and neighbours are calling less often. The relatives continue to grieve and must be allowed to do this at their own pace and in their own time. They will feel great sadness but this is often accompanied by feelings of relief, especially if the illness has been a long and painful one – yet they may also feel guilty because they feel relieved. There are also feelings of guilt about the care they have given: was it adequate? Did they do enough? Was there anything else they might have done? They begin to feel very lonely, especially if they have lost a spouse. The less domesticated man finds it difficult to cope with the housekeeping and he may become depressed and undernourished. The woman finds invitations that were plentiful for her husband and herself coming less and less frequently, and her sense of isolation grows. The elderly daughter with unaccustomed time on her hands may have difficulty in planning the future now that she has the freedom to do so. Here the volunteer can give great help and support if she continues to visit and show an interest.

The death of a child

When a young child dies, the grief and loss is magnified as the parents mourn the young life ended so quickly. They feel extreme guilt that the child is dead and they are alive, and blame themselves for doing something wrong. They may need a great deal of help and support to carry on. Try to prevent them sweeping away all traces of the child: reminders in the days to come will be very precious.

The volunteer's role

Try to encourage families or groups to grieve together. Where the death has come suddenly as part of a large disaster, support groups often form spontaneously and the group sharing of grief is helpful. Talking about the loved one, looking at photographs, remembering all the happy times together is very therapeutic. Make sure parents or relatives do not exclude the children, however young, as they too experience the sense of bereavement and loss, and they too need to grieve, although they may not fully understand the circumstances.

The volunteer can, of course, be of the greatest help when the bereavement has left one person alone – perhaps a husband, wife or ageing daughter. They have no one to talk to and no one to share in their recollections. Try to introduce them to an organization like Cruse, or to a local lunch club where they can find companionship. Any time you yourself can give is time well spent. Remember particularly the first anniversary of the death: they might appreciate you going with them to the graveside, or simply visiting for a chat. Grief passes slowly, slower for some than others, and anniversaries of births, deaths and weddings are particularly painful. Do all you can to help at such times. This is one field where the volunteer has the opportunity to show a real caring spirit and to give her time and support for as long as it is needed.

APPENDIX I: NORMAL DEVELOPMENT –
BIRTH TO FIVE YEARS

The normal healthy infant has a clear firm skin, bright eyes, breathes through his nose with his mouth closed, and is contented, active and happy. He is ready for his meals, enjoys them and digests them easily. He sleeps well and shows recognizable signs of physical and mental development.

All children are individuals and there is considerable variation between them depending on character, surroundings and heredity, and their cultural and social environment. There are no hard and fast rules, but the study of hundreds of babies has made it possible to map out average times at which a certain degree of development is reached. This does not mean, however, that a baby is abnormal if he develops later than the times suggested.

Progress is often irregular, in particular weight gain, and mothers worry unnecessarily because a week or two passes without any increase. If the child appears healthy there is no need for concern and a regular visit to the family practitioner or child health clinic will ensure the child's development is adequately supervised.

PHYSICAL DEVELOPMENT

Height
At birth the baby usually measures about 50cm (20in); at one year 72.5cm (29in); during the next year or two he will grow about 10cm (4in) a year. After this the rate of growth slows to about 5cm (2in) a year. Growth may be slower in an undernourished child or if there has been illness. The child reaches approximately half his adult stature by the end of the second year.

Weight
A baby will approximately double his birth weight by three months and treble it by a year. For example, a baby weighing 3.2kg (7lb) at birth will weigh 6.4kg (14lb) at three months and 9.6kg (21lb) at one year. After this the gain is slightly less: about 3.6kg (8lb) in the second year, 2.2kg (5lb) in the third, and 1.8kg (4lb) in the fourth and fifth. By his fifth birthday he will weigh about 19kg (42lb). This will vary a great deal: provided the baby is happy and healthy there is no cause for worry.

Teeth
All the first dentition are present in the gums at birth, being formed whilst the baby is growing in the uterus. For this reason it is important that the expectant mother's diet

AVERAGE WEIGHT AND HEIGHT OF INFANTS

Birth	3.2kgs	(7lb)	50cm	(20in)
1 Year	9.5kgs	(21lb)	72.5cm	(29in)
2 Years	12.5kgs	(28lb)	82.5cm	(32in)
3 Years	15kgs	(33lb)	92.5cm	(36in)
4 Years	16.5kgs	(36lb)	100cm	(39in)
5 Years	19kgs	(42lb)	105cm	(42in)

includes adequate amounts of calcium and vitamin D, which are needed for the healthy growth of bones and teeth: this is why she is encouraged to take at least one pint of milk in some form each day. The teeth erupt at different times, but this varies a great deal; some babies are born with one tooth and some do not cut their first tooth until the fifteenth month. The average time is about the seventh month and most children have their full set of twenty teeth by the middle of the second year.

Eruption of teeth

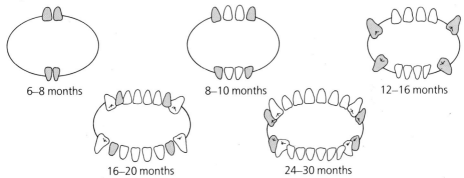

6–8 months   8–10 months   12–16 months

16–20 months   24–30 months

MENTAL DEVELOPMENT

In the same way as bodily growth varies, so do character, temperament and intelligence. A placid baby tends to sleep for long periods and as he grows he will accept life around him quietly. The excitable baby may sleep only for one or two hours at a time, and later when he begins to crawl around will be in and out of everything.

Children thrive best when they feel secure, and when they know they have the protection of adults. Many problems of childhood arise from a lack of security if the child feels unloved and unwanted. These feelings commonly arise with the arrival of a new baby, especially when the mother has gone into hospital and arrives home with a baby which takes up most of her time. The older child needs a great deal of love and involvement if he is not to be jealous. His help in preparing for the baby and caring for him once he has arrived goes a long way to solving this problem. Another occasion when the child feels unwanted is if he has to be admitted to hospital for any reason and he is cut off from all he knows and loves. Again, careful preparation, a favourite toy to go with him and constant visiting by the parents do much to help.

Children learn by listening and watching and by imitating. A child who sees his parents washing their hands before meals, or cleaning their teeth afterwards, will often do likewise without instruction. Similarly, if no one spends time talking with him, he can never imitate the sounds which will eventually make speech; and his facility with words in later life depends very much on the kind of conversation he hears at home. The family that converses in short sentences or single words may produce a child who finds learning difficult at school, because he is not accustomed to listening to the longer sentences the teacher uses.

Children should be allowed to develop naturally. No child should be forced to sit up or to stand until he shows signs of trying on his own. If left to themselves children tend to know what they should do and when. They need to be given the chance to explore the environment for themselves and through this to develop their individuality and mental ability.

MILESTONES

	Activity	Intelligence	Approximate weigh
One to two months	The infant sleeps most of the 24 hours and, when awake, waves his arms and legs in an aimless fashion. He will grasp things when they are put in his hand. He can hold his head erect for a few seconds.	He has a different cry to express pain or hunger. He cannot see clearly at first but will fix his eyes on his mother and by six to eight weeks will smile and follow a bright light.	He gains up to about 180g (6oz) a week. A baby weighing 3.2kg (7lb) at birth will weigh about 4.5kg (10lb) at two months.
Three to four months	The infant holds his head steady when held in the arms. When he lies on his back he may try to roll over. He plays with his fingers and begins to follow moving objects with his eyes.	He makes noises and recognizes his mother.	He gains about 180–240g (6–8oz) a week, and at four months will weigh about 6.4kg (14lb).
Six months	The movements are now more coordinated and purposeful. The child will reach out and grasp toys with his hands and will play with his toes. He can now sit without support for a short while.	He recognizes friends as well as parents and shows pleasure by smiles or laughter and displeasure by frowns or crying.	7kg (15lb) or more.
Nine months	Sits up alone, crawls and may be trying to pull himself up. Will be able to reach forward when sitting up without losing his balance. Can be taught to crawl towards things he wants and to wave his hands. Begins to use his index finger to poke into holes.	He may say one or two words such as "Mum" and "Dad", and understands the meaning of obedience.	Gaining about 480g (1lb) a month.
Twelve months	He may have learnt to walk but may need a guiding hand or will hold on to things. Can pull himself up on furniture. Can hold a crayon, and plays with bricks.	He will be saying two or three words or more and understands clearly the meaning of "yes" and "no". Will look at simple picture books.	He is gaining 240–360g (8–12oz) a month and at one year weighs between 9.5 and 10kg (21–22lb).

Sleep	Fontanelle/Teeth/ Diet	Suitable toys
	Fontanelle: He has a soft diamond-shaped area on the top of the head called the anterior fontanelle, and a smaller triangular one at the back of the head called the posterior fontanelle, which closes soon after birth.	From about five weeks he will watch mobiles suspended above him.
20 hours.	**Diet:** Weaning is begun at about four months. Small amounts of solid food are given at first to introduce the baby to new flavours and textures.	Anything that makes a noise, and is lightweight and unbreakable; perhaps a tin filled with beans and carefully sealed.
18 hours.	**Fontanelle:** The soft area in the middle of the skull is now smaller. **Teeth:** There may be one or two front teeth by about the end of the sixth month. **Diet:** Still breast-fed or having a bottle but has now been having solid foods for about two months.	He will love looking in a mirror near – but never in – his cot. Any toy with crevices, holes or handles for him to explore. Musical boxes will please him.
17 hours.	**Teeth:** Approximately six, four of which will be the two upper and two lower front teeth. **Diet:** Drinking out of a cup and eating most foods suitable for a baby of his age, provided they are sieved, mashed or minced.	Any toy with knobs and buttons which he can push, or which can be made to make a noise. Washable soft toys.
16 hours.	**Teeth:** Eight to ten in number.	Large bricks, cotton reels, spoon and a tin or a saucepan which he enjoys banging about; toys that rattle or can be pushed; plastic ducks or boats that can float in the bath. Toy dogs, trains, etc. that can be pulled on a string.

MILESTONES CONTINUED

	Activity and intelligence	Approximate weight
Eighteen months	He walks easily and steadily, runs and enjoys pushing or pulling wooden toys on wheels. Will be able to balance while he bends to pick something up. Has learned turning and screwing movements. Will be able to wash his hands and perhaps walk upstairs. Prefers to play alone or with an adult rather than with other babies of his own age. He feeds himself with a spoon and says a few words.	10.5–11.5kg (23–25lb).
Two years	He runs, throws a ball and is able to climb on a stool. Talks well, names familiar objects and will listen to stories and nursery rhymes. Instead of unformed scribbling he now makes up and down strokes with a crayon. He is just beginning to play with other children and has now learnt clean habits.	12.5kg (28lb).
Three years	He plays simple games with other children, runs quickly, jumps, sings, dances, rides a tricycle. He will walk upstairs with a foot on each stair, but will put both feet on the same stair coming down. He will stand for a few seconds on one foot. Points out familiar objects, and will copy a circle. Answers simple questions and carries out simple errands. Helps to wash and dress himself, perhaps buckling his own sandals, and will help parents in simple household tasks. Talks about his own activities.	15kg (33lb).
Four to five years	A child at this stage is more independent and is able to hold his own with other children. He prefers to be with children of his own age during most of the day and needs companionship. He has knowledge of the use of common articles between which he differentiates without difficulty. Thoroughly enjoys motion songs to music and will play happily with sand, water or Plasticine. He will make simple drawings with coloured pencils or crayons.	At four years 16.5kg (36lb); at five years 19kg (42lb).

Sleep	Fontanelle/Teeth/Diet	Suitable toys
14 hours.	**Fontanelle:** The soft area on the head is now closed. **Teeth:** 12 to 16 in number.	Somewhat bigger washable soft toys of definite shape, such as a boy, a girl, a dog, a cat. Building beakers, nesting cubes, hammer pegs; he will be able to build a tower of bricks. He will like trucks and large wooden toys on four wheels, but they should be stable so they do not cause him to fall over.
14 hours.	**Teeth:** 18 to 20 in number. First visit to the dentist about now.	Simple put-together toys such as screw toys, toys with wooden nuts and bolts, jigsaws with not more than ten to twelve pieces, dolls, crayons and paper, picture dominoes. Wheelbarrow, wooden train, wooden truck or roller.
12 to 14 hours.	**Teeth:** 20 in number.	Hammer pegs, mosaics, building bricks. Modelling clay and Plasticine fulfil the urge to create. A Wendy house or discarded play-pen and rug, a miniature nurse's uniform or policeman's helmet give scope for imagination.
12 hours.	**Diet:** He is now eating the same foods as the rest of the family.	Large jigsaws, painting, drawing pencils, building meccano, magnetic letters and numbers. Children of this age enjoy group activity as well as solitary play; they love climbing frames, sandpits, swings and slides, and playing with pets such as cats and dogs – although a parent or adult will need to supervise.

APPENDIX II

COMMUNICABLE DISEASES

COMMON INFECTIOUS DISEASES

Disease Incubation period	Signs and Symptoms	Isolation of patient	Availability of immunization
Chickenpox 17–21 days	Elevated temperature; dark red, irritating groups of spots which appear every 3–4 days	Isolate for 7 days from onset of rash	No
Gastroenteritis Depends on cause	Diarrhoea, vomiting, abdominal pain	Isolate	No
German measles (rubella) 14–21 days	Slightly raised temperature; enlarged glands at the back of the neck; rash behind the ears spreading to the face and body	Keep away from school for approximately one week. Other children may continue at school but expectant mothers should not work at the school unless vaccinated	Available for girls aged 11–14
Influenza 2–3 days	Elevated temperature; sore throat, runny nose, cough, hoarse voice, headache, aching joints	Keep away from school until recovered	Yes – in special circumstances
Measles (morbilli) 10–14 days	Elevated temperature; runny nose, cough, inflamed eyes; white (Koplik's) spots in the mouth; blotchy red rash behind the ears, spreading to the face and body	Keep away from school until doctor advises return	Yes
Mumps (infective parotitis) 17–21 days	Elevated temperature; swelling and pain in glands at the side of the face; stiff neck and jaw; earache	Keep away from school	No
Whooping cough (pertussis) 6–18 days	Slight rise in temperature; runny nose; slight cough, then a convulsive cough which ends with a gasping "whoop"; vomiting may occur	Isolate whilst child is infectious. Keep away from school until doctor advises return	Vaccination available for children under 3

CHILD IMMUNIZATION

Age	Immunization against:
3 months	Diphtheria Whooping cough Tetanus Poliomyelitis (oral)
5–6 months	Diphtheria Whooping cough Tetanus Poliomyelitis (oral)
9–11 months	Diphtheria Whooping cough Tetanus Poliomyelitis (oral)
12–24 months	Measles
5 years	Diphtheria (booster) Tetanus (booster) Poliomyelitis (oral; booster)
Girls aged 10–14 years	German measles
Girls and boys aged about 13 years	Tuberculosis
School leavers aged about 15–19 years	Tetanus Poliomyelitis (oral)

TRAVELLERS' INFORMATION

Travellers abroad should consult their family practitioner about the protection they require for individual countries.

* Immunization is available at special centres only, for example British Airways and certain infectious diseases hospitals.

Disease	Dose and timing	Protection
Cholera	2 doses 4–6 weeks apart	3–6 months
Hepatitis A	1 dose (normal immunoglobulin)	3 months
Malaria	Tablets before, during and 4 weeks after visit	Only whilst taking tablets
Poliomyelitis	3 doses at monthly intervals	10 years
*Rabies	3 doses separated by 1 month and 1 year	1–2 years
Tetanus	3 doses separated by 6–9 weeks and 6–9 months	5–7 years
Typhoid	2 doses 4–6 weeks apart	3 years
*Yellow fever	1 dose	10 years

APPENDIX III

CONVERSION TABLES

The bold figures in the central column can be read to left or right in each case: for example 35°C equals 95°F, while 35°F equals 2°C.

TEMPERATURE

Centigrade		Fahrenheit
2	**35**	95
4	**40**	104
7	**45**	113
10	**50**	122
13	**55**	131
16	**60**	140
18	**65**	149
21	**70**	158
24	**75**	167
27	**80**	176
32	**90**	194
38	**100**	212

VOLUME

Litres		Pints
0.28	**0.50**	0.88
0.43	**0.75**	1.32
0.57	**1**	1.76
0.71	**1.25**	2.20
0.85	**1.50**	2.64
0.99	**1.75**	3.08
1.14	**2**	3.52
1.42	**2.50**	4.40
1.70	**3**	5.28

LENGTH

Metres		Yards
0.91	**1**	1.09
1.83	**2**	2.19
2.74	**3**	3.28
3.66	**4**	4.38
4.57	**5**	5.47

WEIGHT

Kilograms		Pounds
0.11	**0.25**	0.55
0.23	**0.50**	1.10
0.45	**1**	2.20
0.68	**1.50**	3.31
0.91	**2**	4.41
2.27	**5**	11.02

FURTHER READING

Introduction

G. Aves, *The Volunteer in Practice*, The British Red Cross Society

R. E. Bailey, *Volunteers in Hospital*, St John Ambulance Brigade

P. Barefoot and G. Cunningham, *Community Services – The Health Worker's A–Z*, Faber & Faber

D. Gunn, *A Background to Community Care*, The British Red Cross Society

V. Henderson, *The Nature of Nursing*, Macmillan, New York

N. Kohner, *Caring at Home*, Kings Fund

M. Ward, *A Survey of the Health and Social Services*, The British Red Cross Society

J. Wilson, *Caring Together: Guidelines for Carers' Self-Help and Support Groups*, Kings Fund.

Comfort and Mobility

Handling the Handicapped, Woodhead-Faulkner in association with the Chartered Society of Physiotherapy

People in Wheelchairs, The British Red Cross Society.

Washing and Bathing

Handling the Handicapped, Woodhead-Faulkner in association with the Chartered Society of Physiotherapy.

Clothing

P. Jay, *Help Yourselves* (chapter 4), Ian Henry Publications

Catalogue of Clothing, Disabled Living Foundation

Clothing for the Handicapped Child, Disabled Living Foundation.

Eating and Drinking

A. M. Brown, *Practical Nutrition for Nurses*, Heinemann

Food Additives – A Balanced Approach, Ministry of Agriculture, Fisheries and Food

A Guide to Healthy Eating, Health Education Authority

P. Jay, *Help Yourselves* (chapter 5), Ian Henry Publications

Playing Cards, British Diabetic Association.

Elimination

R. C. L. Fenely and J. P. Blannin, *Incontinence*, Churchill Livingstone, Patient's Handbook 18

D. Mandelstam, *Incontinence*, Heinemann

Notes on Incontinence, Advisory Service, Disabled Living Foundation.

Body Temperature

Warmth in Winter, Health Education Authority/Age Concern.

Communication

P. Jay, *Help Yourselves* (chapter 10), Ian Henry Publications

D. Ritchie, *Stroke – A Diary of Recovery*, Faber & Faber.

Recovery and Rehabilitation

Door to Door, Department of Transport (Freepost, South Ruislip, Middlesex HA4 0NZ)

Plaster of Paris Technique, Smith and Nephew

Sick or Disabled? A Guide to Benefits, Leaflet FB28, Department of Health and Social Security (HMSO).

Recreational Activities

G. Aves, *The Volunteer in Practice*, The British Red Cross Society

Leisure Activities, Disabled Living Foundation.

Learning and Re-Learning

G. Aves, *The Volunteer in Practice*, The British Red Cross Society

J. Carr, *Helping the Handicapped Child: A Step by Step Guide to Everyday Problems*, Penguin Books

T. Griffiths, *Enjoy Your Retirement*, David and Charles

D. M. Jeffree, R. McConkey, S. Hewson, *Let Me Play*, Human Horizons Series

S. Kastein, I. Spaulding, B. Scharf, *Raising the Young Blind Child, A Guide for Parents and Educators*, Human Sciences Press, U.S.A.

K. M. G. Keddie, *Action with the Elderly*, Pergamon Press

R. Lear, *Play Helps*, Heinemann

W. Loving, *A Lively Retirement*, Queen Anne Press

M. R. Marshall, *Parents of the Handicapped Child*, Julia MacRae Books

B. Weller, *Helping Sick Children Play*, Bailliere Tindall

J. A. Muir-Gray, *Better Health in Retirement*, Age Concern

Retiring? Your Pension and Other Benefits, Leaflet FB6, Department of Health and Social Security (HMSO).

The Patient Who is Dying

D. Gunn, *A Background to Community Care*, (Bereavement), The British Red Cross Society

Help When Someone Dies: A Guide to Benefits, Leaflet FB29, Department of Health and Social Security (HMSO)

Red Cross Guide to Welfare (Visiting and Counselling; Reactions to Disaster), The British Red Cross Society

P. Speck, *Loss and Grief in Medicine*, Bailliere Tindall

What to do when Someone Dies, Consumers' Association.

USEFUL ADDRESSES

Comfort and Mobility

The British Red Cross Society Medical Loans Departments (equipment loans): contact nearest branch

The Chartered Society of Physiotherapy (produces leaflets to help prevent back strain or injury) 14 Bedford Row, London WC1R 4ED, 01-242 1941

Disabled Living Foundation, 380–384 Harrow Road, London W9 2HU, 01-289 6111

Muscular Dystrophy Group of Great Britain, Nattrass House, 35 Macaulay Road, London SW4 0QP, 01-720 8055

Rehabilitation Engineering Movement Advisory Panels, 25 Mortimer Street, London W1N 8AB, 01-637 5400

The Royal Association for Disability and Rehabilitation (RADAR), 25 Mortimer Street, London W1N 8AB, 01-637 5400

St Andrew's Ambulance Medical Aids Scheme (equipment loans), St Andrew's House, Milton Street, Glasgow G4 0HR

St John Ambulance Medical Loans Departments (equipment loans): contact nearest branch

The Spastics Society, 12 Park Crescent, London W1N 4EQ, 01-636 5020.

Washing and Bathing

Disabled Living Foundation, 380–384 Harrow Road, London W9 2HU, 01-289 6111

The Royal Association for Disability and Rehabilitation (RADAR), 25 Mortimer Street, London W1N 8AB, 01-637 5400.

Clothing

Disabled Living Foundation, Clothing Advisory Service, 380–384 Harrow Road, London W9 2HU, 01-289 6111.

Eating and Drinking

BACUP (British Association of Cancer United Patients), Information Service, 121–123 Charterhouse Street, London EC1M 6AA, 01-608 1661

British Diabetic Association, 10 Queen Anne Street, London W1M 0BD, 01-323 1531

Disabled Living Foundation, 380–384 Harrow Road, London W9 2HU, 01-289 6111

Marie Curie Cancer Care, 28 Belgrave Square, London SW1X 8QG, 01-235 3325.

Elimination

Colostomy Welfare Group, 38–39 Eccleston Square, London SW1V 1PB, 01-828 5175

Ileostomy Association, Amblehurst House, Black Scotch Lane, Mansfield, Nottinghamshire NG18 4PF, 0623 28099.

Breathing

BOC Ltd (British Oxygen), The Priestley Centre, 10 Priestley Road, The Surrey Research Park, Guildford, Surrey GU2 5XY, 0483 579857

Communication

British Deaf Association, 38 Victoria Place, Carlisle, Cumbria CA1 1HU, 0228 48844

Chest, Heart and Stroke Association, Tavistock House North, Tavistock Square, London WC1H 9JE, 01-387 3012

MIND (National Association for Mental Health), 22 Harley Street, London W1N 2ED, 01-637 0741

Royal National Institute for the Blind, 224 Great Portland Street, London W1N 6AA, 01-388 1266

Royal National Institute for the Deaf, 105 Gower Street, London WC1E 6AH, 01-387 8033

Samaritans: for 24-hour telephone numbers, see local telephone directory.

Recreational Activities

James Galt & Co., Customer Services, Brookfield Road, Cheadle, Cheshire SK8 2PN, 061-428 8511

PHAB (youth clubs and holidays for the physically handicapped and able-bodied), Tavistock House North, Tavistock Square, London WC1H 9HX, 01-388 1963

The British Talking Book Service, Mount Pleasant, Wembley, Middlesex HA0 1RR, 01-903 6666.

Learning and Re-Learning

Age Concern, Bernard Sunley House, 60 Pitcairn Road, Mitcham, Surrey CR4 3LL, 01-640 5431

Counsel and Care for the Elderly, 131 Middlesex Street, London E1 7JF, 01-621 1624

Help the Aged, 16–18 St James's Walk, London EC1R 0BE, 01-253 0253

I Can: Invalid Children's Aid Nationwide, 198 City Road, London EC1V 2PH, 01-608 2462

MENCAP, National Centre, 123 Golden Lane, London EC1Y 0RT, 01-253 9433

Play Matters: The National Toy Libraries Association, 68 Churchway, London NW1 1LT, 01-387 9592

The Pre-Retirement Association of Great Britain and Northern Ireland, 19 Undine Street, Tooting, London SW17 8PP, 01-767 3225

Remploy Ltd (the industrial company set up to give meaningful employment to disabled people), 415 Edgware Road, Cricklewood, London NW2 6LR, 01-452 8020.

The Patient Who is Dying

BACUP (British Association of Cancer United Patients), Information Service, 121–123 Charterhouse Street, London EC1M 6AA, 01-608 1661

Cruse – Bereavement Care, Cruse House, 126 Sheen Road, Richmond, Surrey TW9 1UR, 01-940 4818

Hospice Information Service, St Christopher's Hospice, 51–59 Lawrie Park Road, Sydenham, London SE2 9DZ, 01-778 9252

Marie Curie Cancer Care, 28 Belgrave Square, London SW1X 8QG, 01-235 3325.

INDEX

ACKNOWLEDGMENTS

The text of **Caring for the Sick** was prepared from material written by Rosemary Bailey, M.A., Dip. Ed., RNT, MTD, the former Director of Nursing Education, Hampstead Health District, and a member of St John Ambulance for 34 years and their Chief Nursing Officer from 1972 to 1987.

Editorial Committee
St John Ambulance: Miss R. Bailey, M.A., Dip. Ed., RGN, RNT, MTD
St Andrew's Ambulance Association: Mrs E. Pinkerton, RGN .
The British Red Cross Society: Miss M. Baker, BA, MIHE; Mrs B. Hutchinson, RGN, RNT

Senior Editor   Jemima Dunne
Editor   Sarah Bevan
Designers   Alun Jones and Michelle Stamp of Crucial Books, London
Managing Editor   Daphne Razazan
Art Director   Anne-Marie Bulat

Illustrators
Kuo Kang Chen, Coral Mula, Mary Tomlin

Photography
Geoff Dann

Typesetting
Goodfellow & Egan

Reproduction
Colourscan

Dorling Kindersley would like to thank: Eleanor Fison, Ann Lilley, Denise Loach, Philip Lord, Eric Ploss, Maggie Ramsay, Shaun Seely, Sam Smith and members of staff at Dorling Kindersley for acting as models for the photographs; Miss Helen Gribble; and the staff and children of Oadby Red Cross Toy Library for their generous help.